Applied Psychology Readings

Peter Macaulay · Lee-Ming Tan
Editors

Applied Psychology Readings

Selected Papers from the Singapore Conference on Applied Psychology 2022

Springer

Editors
Peter Macaulay
College of Health, Psychology and Social Care
University of Derby
Derby, UK

Lee-Ming Tan
East Asia Research
Singapore, Singapore

ISBN 978-981-99-2612-1   ISBN 978-981-99-2613-8 (eBook)
https://doi.org/10.1007/978-981-99-2613-8

This Springer imprint is published by the registered company Springer Nature Singapore Pte Ltd.
The registered company address is: 152 Beach Road, #21-01/04 Gateway East, Singapore 189721, Singapore

SCAP Advisory Board

Conference Chair

Committee Members

Supporting Journals

Jurnal Psikologi Ulayat: Indonesian Journal of Indigenous Psychology (JPU)
Jurnal Psikologi
Buletin Psikologi
RUDN Journal of Psychology and Pedagogics
Gadjah Mada Journal of Professional Psychology
Gadjah Mada Journal of Psychology
Psihologija Journal

Conference Sponsors

Australian Association of Psychologists Inc
Australian Aviation Psychology Association (AAvPA)
Bulgarian Psychological Society
Colegio Colombiano de Psicólogos
Lithuanian Psychological Association
Mongolian Psychologists Association
Serbian Psychological Society
Sociedade Brasileira de Psicologia

Conference Organizer

East Asia Research

East Asia Research (EAR)

Established in Singapore in 2015, East Asia Research (EAR) envisions to be the gateway to improving lives and enhancing productivity in Asia through promoting cross-geographical exchange of ideas and knowledge in various faculties. This will be achieved through the dissemination of knowledge from the Asia-focused research conferences and publications by EAR.

EAR academic conferences provide a meaningful platform for researchers, post-graduates, academicians, and industry practitioners to share unique insights and drive innovation. This is a great opportunity for expanding contact networks beyond a singular field and kick-starting a strategic collaboration. Such partnership can bridge the resources and expertise of multiple disciplines to spearhead pioneer movements, giving rise to breakthroughs in long-standing issues.

Preface

The 2022 Singapore Conference on Applied Psychology, organized by East Asia Research and supported by Singapore University of Technology and Design and the University of Derby, was held on 8–9 December 2022. Researchers and practitioners from many fields of applied psychological research and practice presented on a range of recent innovations, trends, practical challenges, and solutions adopted in the field of Applied Psychology, with a special focus on psychological well-being. Presentations were given from academics and practitioners in over 10 countries and keynote presentations were given by Dr. Carrie Childs from the University of Derby, who presented on 'Experiences of Relations and Connections in 12 Step Programmes for "Sex Addiction"', along with Dr. Yow Wei Quin from Singapore University of Technology and Design, who presented on 'A Lifespan Perspective of Psychological Well-Being—The Moderating Role of Age in Perceived Well-Being' and Dr. Samuel Chng from Singapore University of Technology and Design, who presented on 'Cities, Complexity, Psychology'.

This book includes 8 papers submitted and accepted for special publication following a peer-review process supported by academics at the University of Derby, co-ordinated by Dr. Peter Macaulay. The papers selected for publication cover an exciting and diverse range of empirical studies and discussion in the field of applied psychology.

The 2023 Singapore Conference on Applied Psychology 2023 will be held on the 7–8 December 2023 in Singapore.

Derby, UK
SCAP 2022

Dr. Peter Macaulay

Contents

About the Editors

Dr. Peter Macaulay He is a Lecturer in Psychology in the School of Psychology, University of Derby, UK. His main research interests lie within the area of social developmental psychology. In particular, his work focuses on the perceptions and experiences of cyberbullying, face-to-face bullying, and bystander intervention. Dr Macaulay's research explores how teachers and young people perceive and respond to cyberbullying in the school environment. His research also examines how young people perceive personal and situational factors in bullying, and how this may impact on their bystander intervention. Dr Macaulay regularly publishes in peer-reviewed journals, and conducts some of his work on anti-bullying interventions in schools.

Mr. Lee-Ming Tan He is the founder of East Asia Research and he obtained his Master of Applied Finance from The University of Adelaide. He is deeply interested in how humans function and react with each other. An insight into how people's minds think and how they work together is invaluable in just about every field. Outside of work, Anthony Tan enjoys outdoor activities and the occasional computer game.

Risk and Protective Factors of Internalizing and Externalizing Symptoms Among Mongolian Adolescents

Altantsetseg Badrakh, Mandukhai Ganbat, Byambajargal Shijir, Togtuunaa Ider, Nandin-Erdene Bayarmagnai, Ganzul Bazarragchaa, Khosgarig Altantsatsralt, and Mandakhbayar Nemekh

Abstract Although internalizing and externalizing symptoms are common among Mongolian adolescents, the risk and protective factors of these symptoms are less investigated in this population. This study explored depression, anxiety, eating-related difficulty, self-harming, bullying, smoking, and alcohol drinking among Mongolian adolescents in relation to the individual, family, and peer-school factors. 1667 adolescents participated through an online platform, and the cross-sectional data analysis was performed on SPSS .25. As hypothesized, parental abuse, peer pressure, and bullying victimization positively predicted all internalizing and externalizing symptoms or were the shared risk factors. Parental emotional neglect positively predicted only self-harming. In contrast, protective factors varied regarding each symptom. Females exhibited more internalizing symptoms, and males exhibited more externalizing symptoms, except for alcohol drinking. Significant age and locational differences were found that older adolescents and those from Ulaanbaatar city were at higher risk to exhibit internalizing and externalizing symptoms. The implication of these results and the future directions are discussed.

Keywords Internalizing and externalizing symptoms · Risk and protective factors · Mongolian adolescents

1 Introduction

Healthy development during adolescence is crucial as it largely determines their later life quality (e.g., Alderman et al., 2019). Yet many adolescents around the world are experiencing internalizing symptoms such as depression and anxiety (Chi et al., 2018;

A. Badrakh · M. Ganbat (✉) · B. Shijir · T. Ider · N.-E. Bayarmagnai · G. Bazarragchaa · K. Altantsatsralt · M. Nemekh
Optimal NMAX LLC, Ulaanbaatar, Mongolia
e-mail: mandukhai@optimal.mn
URL: https://www.optimal.mn

P. Macaulay and L. Tan (eds.), *Applied Psychology Readings*,
https://doi.org/10.1007/978-981-99-2613-8_1

Grist et al., 2019), self-harming (Asarnow & Mehlum, 2019; Mehlum et al., 2019), eating-related difficulties (Warschburger & Zitzmann, 2018), and the externalizing symptoms such as alcohol drinking and smoking (Montgomery et al., 2020) and bullying (Gaffney et al., 2019). Internalizing symptoms are defined as the emotional discomfort and harmful behaviors that are directed toward one's self whereas externalizing symptoms are the delinquency and harmful behaviors directed toward the outside, and both are usually signs of emotional disturbance and negative reactions to stressful life events (Achenbach et al., 2016). As these symptoms adversely affect the adolescents' wellbeing (Nash & Bowen, 2002), and even result in the tragedy of suicide in some cases (Davaasambuu et al., 2017), it is becoming increasingly important to investigate and understand those symptoms and their risk and protective factors, in the less studied populations such as Mongolia. Mongolia, located in central Asia, is a developing country with a population of 3.45 million (Kemp, 2022). Mongolia went through three major social structure changes, from traditional nomad herders to a socialist society under the influence of the Soviet Union, and to a capitalist, free market society in the early 1990s (Hurst, 2001). Those radical changes and the economic and political instability created massive public stress, and mental and behavioral issues among the population (see Hurst, 2001). Previous studies (e.g., Davaasambuu et al., 2017; Lee et al., 2019) suggest that Mongolian adolescents are suffering from internalizing and externalizing symptoms, yet, there is a lack of research on the associated factors of those symptoms. To develop a successful preventive intervention, it is crucial to identify which risk and protective factors predict each problem at the individual, family, and peer-school level (Bronfenbrenner, 1979). Therefore, this research intended to fill this gap. Broadly defined, risk factors are the conditions that increase the likelihood of emotional and behavioral negative outcomes, whereas protective factors are the conditions that promote successful development and decrease the negative outcomes (Deković, 1999).

Bronfenbrenner's (1979) ecological theory is one of the most influential theories in understanding adolescents' development and argues that the multiple levels of surrounding environments play an important role in adolescents' development. The theory proposes five levels of environment, starting from the most immediate environment, with which the adolescents interact directly, including the contexts such as family, school, and peers, to a larger macrosystem, which indirectly influences the adolescents' development. The main argument is that to understand adolescents' emotional and behavioral outcomes, the environmental effects must be considered, especially the immediate environment. A similar argument was suggested by the problem behavior theory, which states that not only the individual characteristics such as self-concept but also the environmental factors, or the relationship quality with the significant others, particularly family and peers, predict adolescents' internalizing and externalizing symptoms (Jessor, 1987). When adolescents do not have sufficient psychological skills to deal with adverse life events and do not receive adequate emotional support from their significant others, they display their frustration through such symptoms. According to the latest report from UNICEF on adolescents' mental health and wellbeing (Keeley, 2021), 13% of adolescents around the world are experiencing at least one type of internalizing symptom and the most common ones are depression, anxiety, and eating-related difficulties. The result was explained regarding the adolescents' relationship quality with their significant others in the family and school settings. Moreover, the report stated that more comprehensive data is needed especially from less studied countries (such as Mongolia) to fully understand how the environment affects adolescents' wellbeing.

Mongolia is a country of youth and around one in five Mongolians is aged 10–19 (National Statistics' Commission, 2021). Unfortunately, adolescents' internalizing and externalizing symptoms are relatively common in Mongolia. For example, higher prevalence of suicidal thoughts and attempts (i.e., one in three adolescents reported they have seriously considered committing suicide (Badarch et al., 2022)), and a significantly higher prevalence of alcohol drinking (Dashpuntsag et al., 2021) and smoking (Sodnom, 2020). Moreover, Mongolian adolescents were the least happy, but the most anxious and lonely ones compared to the adolescents of other low- and middle-income Asian countries (Lee et al., 2019). However, previous studies in Mongolia tended to either exclusively focus on the prevalence of the internalizing and externalizing symptoms (e.g., Vanchindorj et al., 2017), or target a single symptom such as smoking (Sodnom, 2020), or suicidal ideation (Davaasambuu et al., 2017). Therefore, there is a need for a more comprehensive study that includes various externalizing and internalizing symptoms and their risk and protective factors simultaneously. By filling this gap, this study intended to explore whether the same risk and protective factors would be accountable for different externalizing and internalizing symptoms and to provide some baseline data for further research projects and the relevant prevention and intervention program development in Mongolia.

Although numerous personal and relationship-related factors were found to be accountable for the adolescents' internalizing and externalizing symptoms in the studies from high-income countries, this study decided to target self-concept and life satisfaction as individual-level protective factors, parental physical and verbal abuse, and parental emotional neglect as family-level risk factors, family cohesion as a family-level protective factor, bullying victimization and peer pressure as the peer- and school-level risk factors, and school satisfaction as the peer- and school-level protective factor. These eight factors were selected for two reasons. First, the modifiable nature of these factors may make them more likely to receive attention from the decision-makers, and evolve into prevention and intervention programs. Second, these selected factors significantly predicted suicidal ideation among Mongolian adolescents (Altangerel et al., 2014). Given the fact that several internalizing and externalizing symptoms were predicted by shared risk and protective factors concurrently in previous studies from other countries (see Monahan et al., 2014), the same factors from Altangerel and others' study might have similar effects on other internalizing and externalizing symptoms.

Also, demographic characteristics such as age, gender, and location tend to have a significant effect in exhibiting the internalizing and externalizing symptoms. Particularly, older adolescence was related to an increased level of internalizing and externalizing symptoms such as depression and anxiety (Chen et al., 2020), smoking (Choi et al., 2001), and alcohol drinking (Windle, 2003). Moreover, female adolescents tend to exhibit more internalizing symptoms, while externalizing symptoms tend to be higher among male adolescents (e.g., Cotter et al., 2016). The reason was explained as peer pressure and delinquent peer associations are higher among boys, therefore resulting in more anti-social behaviors than girls. Whereas the more connection-oriented relationships among girls may produce more anxiety and depression over peer rejection and conflict. The effect of Mongolian culture may play role in the gender differences as well. Traditionally, Mongolians value masculinity and powerfulness in men and submissiveness and softness in women (Hurst, 2001; Rarick et al., 2014), and this cultural effect might enlarge the internalizing symptoms among females and externalizing symptoms among males. However, surprisingly, it was also found that while alcohol drinking was common among male adolescents in most countries, no such gender difference was observed among Mongolian adolescents (Azzopardi et al., 2021). Thus, alcohol drinking can be exceptional from the gender differences, and if supported, this can be a sign that alcoholism might have become a normative culture in Mongolia (Dashpuntsag et al., 2021).

Lastly, the impact of locational difference is huge in Mongolia as the lifestyles of the urban city, Ulaanbaatar, and the countryside have a significant difference. Compared to living in the urban city, living in the countryside might be less harmful to mental health and wellbeing as it is closer to nature, sparsely populated, and less polluted (Tillmann et al., 2018). Indeed, according to Davaasambuu et al. (2017), the suicide risk was higher among adolescents living in Ulaanbaatar city than those who live in the countryside. Thus, higher levels of internalizing and externalizing symptoms could be expected those from Ulaanbaatar city. Based on the arguments above, the following hypotheses were developed.

H1: Internalizing and externalizing symptoms would have shared risk and protective factors in the individual, family, and school and peer-related domains.
H2: Age would positively predict both internalizing and externalizing symptoms.
H3: Females would demonstrate higher levels of internalizing symptoms and males would demonstrate higher levels of externalizing symptoms, except for alcohol drinking.
H4: Participants from Ulaanbaatar city would demonstrate higher levels of both internalizing and externalizing symptoms.

2 Methodology

2.1 Participants and Procedure

Adolescents in Mongolia aged 14–19 were invited to participate voluntarily and anonymously through a popular teen social media platform, Positive DADAL, in October 2021. Adolescence is the age period between 10 and 19, according to World Health Organization (2001). However, as this study was carried out during COVID-19 restrictions, online data collection was the most feasible option. The age range was determined as adolescents aged above 13 are allowed to use social media platforms, and 96% of those adolescents use social media daily in Mongolia (Communications & Regulatory Commissions of Mongolia, 2021). Ethical approval was received from the research committee of the School of Social Science of the National University of Mongolia. The online questionnaire was distributed along with the information sheet, informed consent (i.e., parental consent for participants who are below 18 years old), and the debrief. Participants had to obtain consent from their parents and tick the parental consent box located at the bottom of the informed consent page, if they were aged below 18. In the debrief, information was provided on receiving mental health support if they felt distressed during or after the survey. Participants also provided a pseudonym for withdrawal requests. The pseudonym nickname creation was also used to mitigate the threats of bots (Pozzar et al., 2020). As 2105 responses were received, 1667 were included in the data analyses after excluding the incomplete responses (i.e., responses with at least one missing data were treated as incomplete and were removed, therefore, yielding a 79.1% response rate). Among the 1667 participants, 28.9% were 14 years old, 23.9% were 15 years old, 17.7% were 16 years old, 19.6% were 17 years old, 5.5% were 18 years old, and 4.4% were 19 years old. In terms of gender 54.3% were females and 45.7% were males, 69.7% were from Ulaanbaatar city and the remaining 30.3% were from the countryside.

2.2 *Measures*

The original scales were in English. Therefore, a two-way translation was performed from English into Mongolian by the third and fifth authors who are native Mongolian speakers with a proficient level of English, and a back-translation by the first author who is also a native Mongolian speaker and educated in the UK. Smoking and alcohol drinking were assessed by one-item dichotomous questions. We conducted a pilot test with 20 participants to check the cultural adaptation of the translated scales. In the pilot test, some of the respondents complained that the total questionnaire was too long. Moreover, due to the language and cultural differences, some items of the translated scales were repetitive, thus, making the respondents feel confused. Thus, to shorten the number of items, repetitively translated items were excluded. The internal consistencies of the final scales were in the acceptable range for short scales (Streiner, 2003).

Life satisfaction. Diener et al.'s (1985) the Satisfaction with Life Scale assessed general life satisfaction through five items such as "*I am satisfied with my life*" and "*Conditions of my life are excellent*". Responses range from 1 (strongly disagree) to 7 (strongly agree), thus higher scores indicate higher life satisfaction. The internal consistency of the original scale was $\alpha = 0.87$ and the two-month test–retest coefficient was 0.82 (Diener et al., 1985). The internal consistency of this translated scale was $\alpha = 0.76$, or highly consistent.

Self-concept. Self-concept (i.e., beliefs they hold about themselves) was assessed through six dimensions: perceived behavior, anxiety, intellectual status, popularity, physical appearance, and happiness using the Adolescents' Self-concept Short Scale (Veiga & Leite, 2016). The scale includes items such as "*I am good-looking*" and "*It is easy to get along with me*" and responses range from 1 (total disagreement) and 6 (total agreement). Thus, higher scores indicate a more positive self-concept. The original scale has 30 items, and this study used 12 selected items (two items from each dimension). The internal consistencies of the original scale and the translated scale were $\alpha = 0.87$ (Veiga & Leite, 2016) and $\alpha = 0.81$, or both highly consistent.

Parental abuse. Eight selected items from National Child Abuse and Neglect study (Browne et al., 2002) were used to measure parental verbal and physical abuse. For example, "*Do your parents/primary guardian hit you when they are upset?*" and "*At home, do they say bad words to you?*". Answers range from 1 (never) to 5 (all the time), thus higher scores indicate a higher level of parental abuse. The internal consistency was $\alpha = 0.74$, or highly consistent.

Parental emotional neglect. Assessed parental emotional neglect through the 5-item Emotional Needs subscale of the Neglect Scale (Straus et al., 1997), including items such as "*did not comfort me when I was upset*" and "*did not tell me they loved me*". Responses range from 1 (strongly disagree) to 4 (strongly agree). Higher scores indicate a higher level of parental emotional neglect. The internal consistencies of the original scale and the translated scale were $\alpha = 0.89$ (Straus et al., 1997) and $\alpha = 0.84$, or both highly consistent.

Family cohesion. The Family Balanced Cohesion subscale of FACES-IV (Olson, 2011) was used in measuring family supportiveness and togetherness. The scale has seven items such as "*Family members are supportive of each other during difficult times*", and "*Family members consult each other on important decisions*". Responses range from 1 (strongly disagree) to 5 (strongly agree). Higher scores indicate a higher level of family cohesion. The internal consistency of the original subscale ranged from alpha 0.75 to 0.89, a three-week test–retest reliability coefficient ranged from 0.83 to 0.93, and the convergent validity assessment showed that the subscale was strongly correlated (0.89–0.98) with the other theoretically related measures such as Self-Report Family Inventory (Olson, 2011; Tiesel & Olson, 1997). The internal consistency of the translated scale was $\alpha = 0.94$, or highly consistent.

School satisfaction. Participants' school satisfaction was measured by the Relationship with Classmates subscale of the High School Satisfaction Scale (Lodi et al., 2019). The scale has four items such as "*I am satisfied with my friendships with my classmates*". We added two items specifically for the relationship with teachers (e.g., "*I am satisfied with the way my teachers communicate with me*"), and an item for general school satisfaction ("*I am generally satisfied with my school*") as these are another crucial aspect to consider when measuring school satisfaction. Responses range from 1 (not at all) to 5 (extremely). Higher scores indicate a higher level of school satisfaction. The internal consistency of the original subscale was $\alpha = 0.88$, and the concurrent validity coefficient with other standardized scale was 0.72, or highly correlated (Lodi et al., 2019). The internal consistency of this translated version's was $\alpha = 0.77$, or highly consistent.

Peer pressure. The Peer pressure questionnaire (Santor et al., 2000) assessed peer pressure, conformity, and popularity through nine selected items such as "*At times, I ignored some people to get more popular*", "*I often feel pressured to do things I wouldn't normally do*", and "*If my friends are drinking, it would be hard for me to resist*". Answers range from 1 (strongly disagree) to 5 (strongly agree). Thus, higher scores indicate a higher level of peer pressure. The internal consistency of the original scale ranged from alpha 0.69 to 0.91 (Santor et al., 2000). The internal consistency of this version was $\alpha = 0.77$, or highly consistent.

Bullying victimization. Bullying victimization experiences were assessed by the Victim subscale of the Revised Olweus bully/victim questionnaire (Olweus, 1996). The subscale measured physical, emotional, and online bullying through nine items such as "*I was called mean name, was made fun of, and teased in a hurtful way*". Responses range from 1 (this has not happened to me) to 5 (several times a week). Thus, higher scores indicate a higher level of victimization. The psychometric validation has been well received on this measurement. The internal consistency of the victim subscale ranged from alpha 0.86 to 0.91 (Gaete et al., 2021; Hartung et al., 2011), the relationship between self-reported victimization on the subscale and peer nomination was moderate (0.42), and a six-month anonymous follow-up study showed similar counts of self-reported victims (Lee & Cornell, 2009). The internal consistency of the translated version was $\alpha = 0.71$, or highly consistent.

Depression. Depressive symptoms were assessed through a 10-item, depression subscale of the DSM-oriented Youth-Self-Report questionnaire, 11–18 years old version (Achenbach & Rescorla, 2001). Thirteen items such as "*I feel unhappy, sad, and depressed*" and "*I think about killing myself*" were used, with answers ranging from 1 (not true) to 3 (very true). Higher scores indicate higher risk of depression. The convergent validity coefficient tested against the Depression Self-Rating Scale was 0.61 or showed a good correlation (Ivarsson et al., 2002). The internal consistency ranged from alpha 0.80 to 0.90 in published studies (see Begovac et al., 2004; Steinhausen & Metzke, 1998). The internal consistency of this version was $\alpha = 0.89$, or all highly consistent.

Anxiety. Anxious symptoms were assessed through the Anxiety subscale of DSM-oriented Youth-Self-Report questionnaire, 11–18 years old version (Achenbach & Rescorla, 2001). The scale was tested against standardized clinical diagnoses and the results supported its' concurrent validity (Ferdinand, 2008). Nine items such as "*I am nervous or tense*" were used, with answers ranging from 1 (not true) to 3 (very true). Higher scores indicate higher risk of anxiety. The internal consistencies of the original scale and the translated scale were $\alpha = 0.73$ (Ferdinand, 2008) and $\alpha = 0.77$, or both highly consistent.

Eating difficulty. Bulimia, weight, and body-image-related nine items, such as "*I avoid eating when I am hungry*", from the Eating Attitudes Test—short form (Garner et al., 1982) were used. Answers ranged from 1 (never) to 6 (always). Higher scores indicate higher risk of eating difficulty. The internal consistency of the original scale was $\alpha = 0.90$ among at risk group, and the test–retest reliability ranged from 0.84 to

0.89 (Banasiak et al., 2001). The internal consistency of this study's was $\alpha = 0.84$, or highly consistent.

Self-harming. Self-harm inventory (Sansone & Sansone, 2010) explores lifetime intentional self-harming behaviors through items such as "*Have you ever intentionally cut yourself?*". Six selected items—self-cutting, burning, hitting, abusing the medication, making the medical situation worse on purpose, and torturing oneself on purpose—out of the original 22 items were used. The rest of the items were either repetitive or culturally inadaptable. For instance, driving a car and getting employed is illegal for adolescents in Mongolia. Answers range from 1 (never) to 5 (most of the time). Higher scores indicate higher risk of self-harming. The internal consistency of the original scale among non-clinical sample was $\alpha = 0.83$ (Latimer et al., 2009) and this study's was $\alpha = 0.72$, or both highly consistent.

Bullying. The bullying subscale of the Revised Olweus Bully/Victim Questionnaire (Olweus, 1996) was used in measuring the bully-perpetration experiences. Six selected items were included, such as, "*I spread false rumors about him or her and tried to make others dislike him or her*" and "*I bullied him or her with mean or hurtful comments, messages, calls, or pictures, or in any other ways on the Internet*" receiving answers ranging from 1 (never) to 5 (several times a week). Higher scores indicate higher risk of bullying others. The internal consistency ranged between alpha 0.76 and 0.81 in published studies (see Young, 2020) and the internal consistency of this version's was 0.60, or in the acceptable range.

Smoking. Lifetime smoking experience was measured by an item (*Have you ever smoked a cigarette?*), with a yes or no dichotomous answer.

Alcohol drinking. Lifetime alcohol drinking experience was measured by an item (*Have you ever drunk alcohol?*), with a yes or no dichotomous answer.

2.3 Analyses Plan

The analyses were conducted on SPSS .25 (IBM Corp., 2017). After examining the bivariate correlations, a one-way MANOVA was run to examine how age (continuous) would associate with the internalizing and externalizing symptoms (H2). To check the gender and locational differences in internalizing and externalizing symptoms (H3 and H4), t-tests were run for the continuous dependent variables (depression, anxiety, self-harming, eating difficulty, and bullying), and chi-square tests were run for the categorical dependent variables (smoking and alcohol drinking). After that, controlling for the demographic variables (age (continuous), gender (male = 0, female = 1), and location (Ulaanbaatar = 0, countryside = 1) were entered in the first block), linear regressions were conducted for the continuous dependent variables, and logistic regressions were conducted for the categorical dependent variables, to examine the associations between the risk and protective factors and the externalizing and internalizing symptoms (H1).

3 Results

3.1 Bivariate Correlations

All dependent variables correlated with each other positively, as shown in Table 1.

Table 2 shows the protective factors, (i.e., life satisfaction, self-concept, family cohesion, and school satisfaction) positively correlated with each other and negatively correlated with the risk factors, (i.e., parental abuse, parental emotional neglect, peer pressure, and bullying victimization).

Table 3 shows that significant correlations were found between independent variables and dependent variables. The protective factors, (i.e., life satisfaction, self-concept, family cohesion, and school satisfaction) negatively correlated with all of the internalizing and externalizing symptoms, while the risk factors, (i.e., parental

Table 1 Bivariate correlations between dependent variables

	2	3	4	5	6	7
1. Depression	0.708	0.524	0.554	0.213	0.260	0.214
2. Anxiety		0.442	0.430	0.197	0.186	0.134
3. Eating difficulties			0.433	0.171	0.122	0.085
4. Self-harming				0.268	0.246	0.258
5. Bullying					0.206	0.278
6. Smoking						0.400
7. Alcohol drinking						

All correlations were significant at $p < 0.01$

Table 2 Bivariate correlations between independent variables

	2	3	4	5	6	7	8
1. Life satisfaction	0.522	−0.431	−0.473	0.603	0.498	−0.256	−0.236
2. Self-concept		−0.302	−0.442	0.514	0.515	−0.298	−0.258
3. Parental abuse			0.368	−0.518	−0.281	0.245	0.313
4. Parental emotional neglect				−0.695	0.318	0.167	0.156
5. Family cohesion					0.412	−0.244	−0.238
6. School satisfaction						−0.311	−0.302
7. Peer pressure							0.345
8. Bullying victimization							

All correlations were significant at $p < 0.01$

abuse, parental emotional neglect, peer pressure, and bullying victimization experiences) positively correlated with all of the internalizing and externalizing symptoms. All correlations were highly significant.

3.2 *Associations Between Age and Internalizing and Externalizing Symptoms*

A one-way MANOVA test was run as age (14–19 years old) entered as continuous independent variable and the internalizing and externalizing symptoms as continuous dependent variables (i.e., smoking and alcohol drinking were treated as continuous data ranging from 0 (no) to 1 (yes)). Generally, there were significant age differences, $F(40, 7212) = 8.66, p = 0.000$; Wilk's lambda = 0.815, partial eta squared = 0.040, that the adolescents tended to exhibit higher levels of internalizing and externalizing symptoms as they get older, with small effect size. Specifically, significant age differences were found in depression ($F(5) = 10.51, p = 0.000$, partial eta squared = 0.031) with small effect size, anxiety ($F(5) = 3.42, p = 0.004$, partial eta squared = 0.010) with small effect size, self-harming ($F(5) = 2.36$, $p = 0.037$, partial eta squared = 0.007) with very small effect size, bullying ($F(5) = 2.90$, $p = 0.013$, partial eta squared = 0.009) with very small effect size, smoking ($F(5) = 31.08$, $p = 0.000$, partial eta squared = 0.086) with medium effect size, and alcohol drinking ($F(5) = 40.87, p = 0.000$, partial eta squared = 0.110) with medium effect size. That is, the strongest effect size of age was found on alcohol drinking and smoking. No age differences were found for eating difficulties ($F(5) = 1.97, p = 0.080$, partial eta squared = 0.006). Therefore, H2 was partially supported.

3.3 *Gender Differences in Internalizing and Externalizing Symptoms*

To check the hypothesis stating that significant gender differences would be present in internalizing and externalizing symptoms, t-tests and chi-square tests were run. Depression was significantly higher for females (M = 17.49, SD = 9.11), $t(1662) = -13.64, p = 0.000$, than males (M = 11.79, SD = 5.08), with large effect size, $g = 0.75$. Anxiety was significantly higher for females (M = 12.83, SD = 9.11), $t(1640) = -9.85, p = 0.000$, than males (M = 10.31, SD = 5.31), with medium effect size, $g = 0.33$. Eating difficulty was significantly higher for females (M = 5.69, SD = 5.70), $t(1491) = -16.77, p = 0.000$, than males (M = 1.92, SD = 3.32), with large effect size, $g = 0.79$. Self-harming was significantly higher for females (M = 2.10, SD = 2.84), $t(1646) = -5.92, p = 0.000$, than males (M = 1.37, SD = 2.15), with small effect size, $g = 0.28$. As opposed to that, bullying was significantly higher for males (M = 2.09 SD = 2.22), t(1451) = 5.02, $p = 0.000$, than females (M = 1.59, SD =

Table 3 Bivariate correlations between independent and dependent variables

	Life satisfaction	Self-concept	Parental abuse	Parental emotional neglect	Family cohesion	School satisfaction	Peer pressure	Bullying victimization
Depression	−0.590	−0.621	0.434	0.409	−0.517	−0.540	0.349	0.339
Anxiety	−0.436	−0.480	0.333	0.264	−0.359	−0.398	0.315	0.320
Eating difficulties	−0.318	−0.350	0.286	0.196	−0.261	−0.297	0.281	0.232
Self-harming	−0.371	−0.364	0.417	0.220	−0.356	−0.367	0.313	0.354
Bullying	−0.186	−0.132	0.224	0.076	−0.158	−0.222	0.372	0.466
Smoking	−0.176	−0.109	0.175	0.113	−0.156	−0.154	0.264	0.211
Alcohol drinking	−0.223	−0.111	0.152	0.123	−0.155	−0.161	0.196	0.154

All correlations were significant at $p < 0.01$

1.78), with small effect size, $g = 0.25$. Smoking was significantly higher for males (yes = 44.1%, no = 55.9%), $X^2(1, 1667) = 25.61$, $p = 0.000$, than females (yes = 32.1%, no = 67.9%), with small effect size, $\varphi = -0.124$. Lastly, contrary to our expectation, alcohol drinking was significantly higher for females (yes = 49.6%, no = 50.4%), $X^2(1, 1667) = 5.05$, $p = 0.025$, than males (yes = 44.0%, no = 56.0%), with small effect size, $\varphi = 0.055$. Therefore, H3 was partially supported.

3.4 Locational Differences in Internalizing and Externalizing Symptoms

To check the hypothesis that significant locational differences would be present in internalizing and externalizing symptoms, t-tests and chi-square tests were run. Depression was significantly higher for adolescents from Ulaanbaatar (M = 15.29, SD = 9.02), $t(1665) = 2.79$, $p = 0.005$, than adolescents from countryside (M = 13.95, SD = 9.06), with small effect size, $g = 0.14$. Anxiety was significantly higher for adolescents from Ulaanbaatar (M = 11.85, SD = 5.35), $t(1665) = 1.99$, $p = 0.046$, than those from countryside (M = 11.28, SD = 5.43), although the strength of significance was weak and the effect size was small ($g = 0.10$). Self-harming was significantly higher for adolescents from Ulaanbaatar (M = 1.96, SD = 2.72), $t(1665) = 4.65$, $p = 0.000$, than adolescents from countryside (M = 1.32, SD = 2.16), with small effect size, $g = 0.24$. Smoking was significantly higher for adolescents from Ulaanbaatar (yes = 39.6%, no = 60.4%), $X^2(1, 1667) = 6.20$, $p = 0.013$, than adolescents from countryside (yes = 33.1%, no = 66.9%), although the strength of significance was relatively weak and the effect size was small ($\varphi = -0.061$). Alcohol drinking was significantly higher for adolescents from Ulaanbaatar (yes = 51.9%, no = 48.1%), $X^2(1, 1667) = 34.24$, $p = 0.000$, than adolescents from countryside (yes = 36.3%, no = 63.7%), with small effect size, $\varphi = -0.143$. However, no difference was observed for eating difficulty, between adolescents from Ulaanbaatar (M = 4.01, SD = 5.21), $t(1665) = 4.74$, $p = 0.636$, and adolescents from countryside (M = 3.88, SD = 4.90). No difference was also observed for bullying, between adolescents from Ulaanbaatar (M = 1.85 SD = 2.06), $t(1665) = 1.67$, $p = 0.281$, and from countryside (M = 1.73, SD = 1.87). Therefore, H4 was partially supported.

3.5 Associations Between Risk and Protective Factors and Internalizing and Externalizing Symptoms

Adjusting for the demographic covariates (age, gender, and location were entered as covariates in the first step), most of the risk and protective factors significantly predicted the internalizing and externalizing symptoms, although, the strength and significance level of the standardized betas and odds ratios vary. The presence of risk and protective factors in the individual, family, and peer and school domains added a significant amount of explained variance beyond that of the demographic variables in the internalizing and externalizing symptoms, as suggested by the R square changes and F changes (see Table 4).

For depression, life satisfaction, positive self-concept, family cohesion, and school satisfaction were negatively associated with, or decreased the risk of depression, while, parental abuse, peer pressure, and bullying victimization experiences were positively associated with, or increased the risk of depression. In terms of anxiety, the results were similar to the depression with slightly weaker beta values, except for peer pressure and bullying victimization, which had slightly stronger beta values than depression or these factors seemed to have a greater effect on anxiety than on depression. For eating difficulty, life satisfaction, positive self-concept, and school satisfaction were negatively associated with or lowered the risk of eating difficulty. While, parental abuse, peer pressure, and bullying victimization were positively associated with or increased the risk of eating difficulty. Self-harming was significantly predicted by all of the risk and protective factors, except for life satisfaction. Specifically, self-concept, family cohesion, and school satisfaction were negatively associated with or lowered the risk of self-harming, while parental abuse, parental emotional neglect, peer pressure, and bullying victimization were positively associated with or increased the risk of self-harming. Bullying was negatively associated with life satisfaction and school satisfaction, or these two factors decreased the risk of bullying, and positively associated with self-concept, parental abuse, peer pressure, and bullying victimization experiences, or these factors increased the risk of bullying others. Of particular note was that positive self-concept, although a protective factor for other symptoms, increased the risk of bullying, with a relatively small effect. For smoking, parental abuse, peer pressure, and bullying victimization experience predicted to increase the odds of smoking. Lastly, regarding alcohol drinking, life satisfaction predicted a decreased odds of alcohol drinking, while parental abuse, peer pressure, and bullying victimization experiences predicted an increased odds of alcohol drinking. That is to say, some factors predicted few or most of the internalizing and externalizing symptoms (i.e., parental emotional neglect, family cohesion, life satisfaction, self-concept, and school satisfaction), and other factors predicted all of the internalizing and externalizing symptoms simultaneously (i.e., parental abuse, peer pressure, and bullying victimization). Therefore, the H1 was partially supported.

Moreover, after accounting for the risk and protective factors, age still positively predicted depression, anxiety, self-harming, smoking, and alcohol drinking, but no association between age and bullying were found anymore. The female gender predicted increased depression, anxiety, eating difficulty, and self-harming, and the male gender predicted increased bullying and smoking. Location significantly predicted depression, self-harming, and alcohol drinking, in which, adolescents from Ulaanbaatar were more at risk. That is, gender differences in alcohol drinking, and locational differences in anxiety and smoking, or the initial weak significance and small effect sizes found in the t-test and chi-squares, became insignificant after taking into account the risk and protective factors simultaneously.

Table 4 Associations between risk and protective factors and internalizing and externalizing symptoms

	Depression β	Anxiety β	Eating difficulty β	Self-harming β	Bullying β	Smoking Odds ratio	Alcohol drinking Odds ratio	
Step 1								
Control covariates (age, gender, and location) R^2	0.125	0.063	0.135	0.038	0.016			
Step 2								
Demographic factors								
Age (continuous)	0.108***	0.047*	0.006	0.051*	0.006	1.616***	1.638***	
Gender (male = 0, female = 1)	0.199***	0.160***	0.329***	0.087***	−0.105***	0.465***	1.179	
Location (Ulaanbaatar = 0, countryside = 1)	−0.041**	−0.031	−0.016	−0.097***	−0.022	0.861	0.533***	
Individual level factors								
Life satisfaction	−0.165***	−0.135***	−0.059*	−0.054	−0.063*	0.979	0.954**	
Self-concept	−0.303***	−0.254***	−0.145***	−0.112***	0.074**	0.999	1.016	
Family level factors								
Parental abuse	0.119***	0.093***	0.106***	0.227***	0.062*	1.110***	1.062*	
Parental emotional neglect	0.007	0.038	0.013	0.083**	0.051	0.991	1.002	
Family cohesion	−0.058*	−0.008	−0.022	−0.075*	−0.010	0.990	0.998	
Peer and school level factors								
School satisfaction	−0.144***	−0.078**	−0.055*	−0.111***	−0.059*	0.999	0.996	

(continued)

Table 4 (continued)

	Depression β	Anxiety β	Eating difficulty β	Self-harming β	Bullying β	Smoking Odds ratio	Alcohol drinking Odds ratio
Peer pressure	0.092***	0.117***	0.167***	0.111***	0.222***	1.080***	1.056***
Bullying victimization	0.108***	0.144***	0.099***	0.173***	0.357***	1.117***	1.092**
R^2	0.599	0.361	0.298	0.328	0.289		
R^2 change	0.474	0.298	0.163	0.290	0.273		
F change	244.74***	96.66***	47.94***	89.08***	79.31***		

* $p < 0.05$. ** $p < 0.01$. *** $p < 0.001$

4 Discussion

This study was one of the first studies that investigated the risk and protective factors of internalizing and externalizing symptoms among Mongolian adolescents with an aim to clarify whether the individual, family, and peer and school-level factors would predict both the internalizing and externalizing symptoms, and more specifically, whether the internalizing and externalizing symptoms would have shared risk and protective factors. We also explored the age, gender, and locational differences in each symptom.

The findings suggested that three out of four risk factors included in this study, parental abuse, peer pressure, and bullying victimization, could be the shared risk factors as these were positively associated with all of the internalizing and externalizing symptoms, while the parental emotional neglect was associated with only self-harming. That is, exposure to the specific risk factor might lead to different behavioral manifestations in different people depending on the interactions with genetic and other environmental effects (Monahan et al., 2014). Particularly, gender difference may play an important role in exhibiting different symptoms when exposed to common risk factors (gender difference is discussed in detail separately). Moreover, the comorbidities in internalizing and externalizing symptoms (Shi et al., 2020) and the significant correlations found in this study among all of the internalizing and externalizing symptoms (Table 1), show that dramatic interrelatedness occurs not only within the symptom domain but also between the two domains (Papachristou & Flouri, 2020). For instance, in the previous studies, depression was correlated with smoking (Farooqui et al., 2022) and alcohol drinking (Milot-Travers & Mahalik, 2021), and these were mostly explained by the self-medication hypothesis which posits that individuals who suffer from internalizing symptoms tend to use alcohol, tobacco, and other substances to cope with the internal negative experiences (Khantzian, 1997). Depression was also associated with bullying others (Uba et al., 2010), as bullies tend to be vulnerable to mental issues perhaps due to the lack of quality relationships with significant others (Kaltiala-Heino et al., 1999). That is to say, exposure to a specific risk factor might also inflict several internalizing and externalizing symptoms, directly and indirectly.

Furthermore, why parental emotional neglect did not predict most of the symptoms included in this study, despite significant associations with internalizing symptoms (Kealy et al., 2020) and externalizing symptoms (Yang et al., 2021) were found in the wider literature, could be a culture-specific effect. Mongolian parents, similar to other Asian parents, tend not to show verbal and behavioral affection and emotional support to their children, and it is somewhat culturally acceptable (Lui & Rollock, 2013). Culturally, Mongolian parents may focus more on their child's physical needs and accomplishments. However, parental emotional neglect did positively predict self-harming behavior. As emotional dysregulation tends to cause self-harming (Asarnow et al., 2021), the results suggest that Mongolian parents being more emotionally supportive can help deal with the adolescents' problematic behaviors such as self-harming. Yet, it should be taken into account that, other risk factors, specifically parental abuse and bullying victimization experiences predicted self-harming more strongly than parental emotional neglect.

In terms of the protective factors, self-concept and school satisfaction were associated with decreased internalizing and externalizing symptoms except for smoking and alcohol drinking. Life satisfaction was associated with decreased internalizing and externalizing symptoms except for self-harming and smoking. Lastly, family cohesion was associated with decreased depression and self-harming. Generally, smoking and alcohol drinking seems to be determined by different protective factors than those included in this study. Especially, contrary to the previous findings from other countries (Brown et al., 2018; Simantov et al., 2000), none of the protective factors were associated with smoking. It might be that this study explored only the lifetime experience of smoking (i.e., Have you ever smoked a cigarette?), and the protective factors included in this study could be better at predicting current or regular smoking.

However, the findings did support that the protective factors that are associated with the internalizing symptoms are also associated with the externalizing symptoms, to some extent. The only exception was that positive self-concept, although a protective factor for other symptoms, was a risk factor for bullying and which needs to be investigated in detail. As the bivariate correlation coefficient between self-concept and bullying was negative, the positive association in the multiple regression might be due to the potential relationships between self-concept and other independent variables. Further studies are encouraged to investigate the univariate and multivariate effects of self-concept on bullying, in-depth.

Furthermore, demographic variables seem to play an important role in understanding the internalizing and externalizing symptoms. Findings supported that female adolescents in Mongolia are more prone to internalizing symptoms and males are prone to externalizing symptoms, consistent with the wider literature from other countries (e.g., Cotter et al., 2016). This gender difference is commonly explained by the gendered personality characteristics of males and females. The manliness, peer pressure, delinquent peer associations, and less expressive communication among boys may result in more anti-social behaviors such as bullying and smoking, whereas, the connection-oriented relationships among girls may make them sensitive to relational conflicts which may result in more internalizing symptoms such as anxiety. Females also tend to underrate their social competence and attractiveness, thus, putting them at greater risk of internalizing symptoms than males (Hoffmann et al., 2004). Also, the Mongolian cultural effect might be influencing these gender differences. Traditionally, masculine aggressiveness is common among Mongolian males, therefore, male gender-based violence tended to be common (Hurst, 2001; Rarick et al., 2014). Our findings suggest that these gendered dynamics might be still present among Mongolian adolescents, to some extent. However, it does not mean that males do not develop internalizing symptoms such as anxiety, and females do not develop externalizing symptoms such as bullying. Moreover, as hypothesized, alcohol drinking was exceptional as the initial small gender difference became insignificant after adjusting to other factors. That is, adolescents in Mongolia are at risk to engage in alcohol drinking irrespective of their gender, in line with a previous study in Mongolia (Azzopardi et al., 2021).

In line with previous research (Davaasambuu et al., 2017), adolescents from Ulaanbaatar were at greater risk to develop some of the internalizing and externalizing symptoms (depression, anxiety, self-harming, smoking, and alcohol drinking) as living in the urban city is more hazardous to their mental health and wellbeing mainly due to the increased stress level resulted from numerous factors such as pollution and overpopulation (Tillmann et al., 2018). However, it should be noted that the effect sizes of the locational differences were generally small and some of them became insignificant (i.e., anxiety and smoking) after adjusting to other factors, and for some of the symptoms no differences were observed at all (i.e., eating difficulty and bullying). Therefore, the preventive interventions perhaps need to focus on adolescents from both Ulaanbaatar and the countryside, equally.

Lastly, age was another risk factor for some internalizing symptoms (depression, anxiety, and self-harming) and externalizing symptoms (smoking and alcohol drinking), in line with previous studies from other countries (Chen et al., 2020; Windle, 2003). Generally, older adolescents were at higher risk of exhibiting internalizing and externalizing symptoms. Especially, smoking and alcohol drinking were most strongly predicted by age. Moreover, as both alcohol drinking and smoking were associated with parental abuse, peer pressure, and bullying, adolescents in Mongolia may experiment with smoking and alcohol drinking to cope with the internal negative experiences, as suggested by the self-medication hypothesis (Khantzian, 1997). Future studies among Mongolian adolescents are encouraged to examine the interaction between age and smoking or drinking as a coping hypothesis.

5 Limitations

This study has some limitations. First, the cross-sectional data limits the potential one-way causal inference that the risk and protective factors cause the internalizing and externalizing symptoms. The internalizing and externalizing symptoms might be contributing to low-quality familial and peer relationships or lower life and school satisfaction. Future studies are encouraged to test the inferences made in this study through longitudinal data. Second, as data collection was carried out during the COVID-19 pandemic restrictions, there could be pandemic-related effects in our findings (Talevi et al., 2020). Therefore, post-pandemic follow-up study is highly encouraged. Third, this study did not take into account the parents' and teachers' perspectives in quantifying the adolescents' situations. Thus, the results of this study only reflect the adolescents' subjective perspective of their current conditions. Future studies can improve the research design by including parents, teachers, and perhaps peers' perspectives. Fourth, there is a number of factors that could be influencing the Mongolian adolescents' emotional and behavioral outcome that are not included in this study. For example, none of the protective factors that are targeted in this study was a shared protective factor that is associated with all of the symptoms simultaneously. Thus, we recommend future studies in Mongolia include more diverse well-established (in other countries) risk and protective factors. Lastly, this study did not clarify current, regular, or binge smoking and drinking in measuring them. That is, this study cannot distinguish the participants who only experimented with smoking or alcohol drinking a few times from those who smoke and drink frequently. Future studies are recommended to investigate smoking and alcohol drinking in-depth, particularly, by assessing the frequency of engagement and motivations behind the engagements.

6 Implications and Future Directions

This study is one of the first that investigated the common emotional and behavioral risks among Mongolian adolescents in relation to their individual, family, and peer and school-related factors. The main implication of this study is it showed the relevant stakeholders in Mongolia that adolescents' emotional and behavioral problems need to be understood within the surrounding environments and how the relationships with significant others can affect adolescents' wellbeing both positively and negatively. Particularly, this study found parental abuse, peer pressure, and bullying victimization predict both internalizing and externalizing symptoms among Mongolian adolescents. Therefore, the intervention and prevention focusing on those shared risk factors can deal with the number of different emotional and behavioral risks among Mongolian adolescents, concurrently. Moreover, the correlations among the internalizing and externalizing symptoms suggest that preventive interventions focusing on a single symptom may have a cross-over effect on dealing with the other symptoms as well.

To develop an effective risk-focused preventive intervention, future studies are encouraged to investigate the qualitative questions to understand why and due to what factors Mongolian parents might abuse their child or Mongolian adolescents bully or pressure each other, and how they define child abuse, bullying, and peer pressure in the cultural context. Nevertheless, it is recommended to initiate anti-parental abuse, bullying, and peer pressure awareness raising in Mongolia. Also, promoting protective factors such as school satisfaction and positive self-concept might be an effective anti-adolescents' emotional and behavioral risk strategy. Lastly, the relevant stakeholders in Mongolia may take the age, gender, and locational effects found in this study into account in dealing with the adolescents' internalizing and externalizing symptoms.

References

Achenbach, T. M., Ivanova, M. Y., Rescorla, L. A., Turner, L. V., & Althoff, R. R. (2016). Internalizing/externalizing problems: Review and recommendations for clinical and research applications. *Journal of the American Academy of Child & Adolescent Psychiatry, 55*(8), 647–656. https://doi.org/10.1016/j.jaac.2016.05.012

Achenbach, T. M., & Rescorla, L. A. (2001). *Manual for the ASEBA school-age forms & profiles: child behavior checklist for ages 6–18, teacher's report form, youth self-report: an integrated system of multi-informant assessment.* University of Vermont, research center for children youth & families.

Alderman, E. M., Breuner, C. C., Grubb, L. K., Powers, M. E., Upadhya, K., & Wallace, S. B. (2019). Unique needs of the adolescent. *Pediatrics, 144*(6). https://doi.org/10.1542/peds.2019-3150

Altangerel, U., Liou, J. C., & Yeh, P. M. (2014). Prevalence and predictors of suicidal behavior among Mongolian high school students. *Community Mental Health Journal, 50*(3), 362–372. https://doi.org/10.1007/s10597-013-9657-8

Asarnow, J. R., & Mehlum, L. (2019). Practitioner review: Treatment for suicidal and self-harming adolescents–advances in suicide prevention care. *Journal of Child Psychology and Psychiatry, 60*(10), 1046–1054. https://doi.org/10.1111/jcpp.13130

Asarnow, J. R., Berk, M. S., Bedics, J., Adrian, M., Gallop, R., Cohen, J., et al. (2021). Dialectical behavior therapy for suicidal self-harming youth: emotion regulation, mechanisms, and mediators. *Journal of the American Academy of Child & Adolescent Psychiatry, 60*(9), 1105–1115. https://doi.org/10.1016/j.jaac.2021.01.016

Azzopardi, P. S., Hennegan, J., Prabhu, S. M., Dagva, B., Balibago, M. M., Htin, P. P. W., et al. (2021). Key recommendations to strengthen public-private partnership for adolescent health in resource constrained settings: Formative qualitative inquiry in Mongolia, Myanmar and the Philippines. *The Lancet Regional Health-Western Pacific, 15*, 100242. https://doi.org/10.1016/j.lanwpc.2021.100242

Badarch, J., Chuluunbaatar, B., Batbaatar, S., & Paulik, E. (2022). Suicide attempts among school attending adolescents in Mongolia: Associated factors and gender differences. *International Journal of Environmental Research and Public Health, 19*(5), 2991. https://doi.org/10.3390/ijerph19052991

Banasiak, S. J., Wertheim, E. H., Koerner, J., & Voudouris, N. J. (2001). Test-retest reliability and internal consistency of a variety of measures of dietary restraint and body concerns in a sample of adolescent girls. *International Journal of Eating Disorders, 29*(1), 85–89.

Begovac, I., Rudan, V., Skočić, M., Filipović, O., & Szirovicza, L. (2004). Comparison of self-reported and parent-reported emotional and behavioral problems in adolescents from Croatia. *Collegium Antropologicum, 28*(1), 393–401.

Bronfenbrenner, U. (1979). *The ecology of human development: Experiments by nature and design.* Harvard University Press.

Brown, J. M., Anderson Goodell, E. M., Williams, J., & Bray, R. M. (2018). Socioecological risk and protective factors for smoking among active duty US military personnel. *Military Medicine, 183*(7–8), e231–e239. https://doi.org/10.1093/milmed/usx021

Browne, K., Cartana, C., Momeu, L., Paunescu, G., Petre, N., & Tokay, R. (2002). *Child Abuse and neglect in Romanian families: A national prevalence study 2000.* Not Known.

Chen, F., Zheng, D., Liu, J., Gong, Y., Guan, Z., & Lou, D. (2020). Depression and anxiety among adolescents during COVID-19: A cross-sectional study. *Brain, Behavior, and Immunity, 88*, 36. https://doi.org/10.1016/j.bbi.2020.05.061

Chi, X., Bo, A., Liu, T., Zhang, P., & Chi, I. (2018). Effects of mindfulness-based stress reduction on depression in adolescents and young adults: A systematic review and meta-analysis. *Frontiers in Psychology, 9*, 1034. https://doi.org/10.3389/fpsyg.2018.01034

Choi, W. S., Gilpin, E. A., Farkas, A. J., & Pierce, J. P. (2001). Determining the probability of future smoking among adolescents. *Addiction, 96*(2), 313–323. https://doi.org/10.1046/j.1360-0443.2001.96231315.x

Communications and Regulatory Commissions of Mongolia. (2021). *Child safety in the online environment*. http://www.ekids.mn/Home/newsdetail?dataID=22030

Cotter, K. L., Wu, Q., & Smokowski, P. R. (2016). Longitudinal risk and protective factors associated with internalizing and externalizing symptoms among male and female adolescents. *Child Psychiatry & Human Development, 47*(3), 472–485. https://doi.org/10.1007/s10578-015-0580-9

Davaasambuu, S., Batbaatar, S., Witte, S., Hamid, P., Oquendo, M. A., Kleinman, M., et al. (2017). Suicidal plans and attempts among adolescents in Mongolia. *Crisis*. https://doi.org/10.1027/0227-5910/a000447

Dashpuntsag, K., Chandaga, U., Tserennadmid, N., Bat-Ochir, U., Mukhtar, Y., Altankhuyag, G. E., et al. (2021). Awareness and attitudes of Mongolian adolescents and youth toward alcohol consumption and alcohol-related harm. *Addiction & Health, 13*(3), 185. https://doi.org/10.22122/ahj.v13i3.1250

Deković, M. (1999). Risk and protective factors in the development of problem behavior during adolescence. *Journal of Youth and Adolescence, 28*(6), 667–685. https://doi.org/10.1023/A:1021635516758

Diener, E. D., Emmons, R. A., Larsen, R. J., & Griffin, S. (1985). The satisfaction with life scale. *Journal of Personality Assessment, 49*(1), 71–75. https://doi.org/10.1207/s15327752jpa4901_13

Farooqui, M., Shoaib, S., Afaq, H., Quadri, S., Zaina, F., Baig, A., et al. (2022). Bidirectionality of smoking and depression in adolescents: A systemic review. *Trends in Psychiatry and Psychotherapy*, (AheadOfPrint). https://doi.org/10.47626/2237-6089-2021-0429

Ferdinand, R. F. (2008). Validity of the CBCL/YSR DSM-IV scales anxiety problems and affective problems. *Journal of Anxiety Disorders, 22*(1), 126–134. https://doi.org/10.1016/j.janxdis.2007.01.008

Gaete, J., Valenzuela, D., Godoy, M. I., Rojas-Barahona, C. A., Salmivalli, C., & Araya, R. (2021). Validation of the revised Olweus bully/victim questionnaire (OBVQ-R) among adolescents in chile. *Frontiers in Psychology, 12*, 578661. https://doi.org/10.3389/fpsyg.2021.578661

Gaffney, H., Ttofi, M. M., & Farrington, D. P. (2019). Evaluating the effectiveness of school-bullying prevention programs: An updated meta-analytical review. *Aggression and Violent Behavior, 45*, 111–133. https://doi.org/10.1016/j.avb.2018.07.001

Garner, D. M., Olmsted, M. P., Bohr, Y., & Garfinkel, P. E. (1982). The eating attitudes test: Psychometric features and clinical correlates. *Psychological Medicine, 12*, 871–878. https://doi.org/10.1017/S0033291700049163

Grist, R., Croker, A., Denne, M., & Stallard, P. (2019). Technology delivered interventions for depression and anxiety in children and adolescents: A systematic review and meta-analysis. *Clinical Child and Family Psychology Review, 22*(2), 147–171. https://doi.org/10.1007/s10567-018-0271-8

Hartung, C. M., Little, C. S., Allen, E. K., & Page, M. C. (2011). A psychometric comparison of two self report measures of bullying and victimization: Differences by sex and grade. *School Mental Health, 3*(1), 44–57. https://doi.org/10.1007/s12310-010-9046-1

Hoffmann, M. L., Powlishta, K. K., & White, K. J. (2004). An examination of gender differences in adolescent adjustment: The effect of competence on gender role differences in symptoms of psychopathology. *Sex Roles, 50*(11), 795–810. https://doi.org/10.1023/B:SERS.0000029098.38706.b1

Hurst, D. (2001). Violence and the crisis of Masculinity in the USA, Australia and Mongolia. *Development, 44*(3), 99–103. https://doi.org/10.1057/palgrave.development.1110272

IBM Corp. Released 2017. IBM SPSS Statistics for Windows, Version 25.0. Armonk, NY: IBM Corp.

Ivarsson, T., Gillberg, C., Arvidsson, T., & Broberg, A. G. (2002). The youth self-report (YSR) and the depression self-rating scale (DSRS) as measures of depression and suicidality among adolescents. *European Child & Adolescent Psychiatry, 11*(1), 31–37. https://doi.org/10.1007/s007870200005

Jessor, R. (1987). Problem-behavior theory, psychosocial development, and adolescent problem drinking. *British Journal of Addiction, 82*(4), 331–342. https://doi.org/10.1111/j.1360-0443.1987.tb01490.x

Kaltiala-Heino, R., Rimpelä, M., Marttunen, M., Rimpelä, A., & Rantanen, P. (1999). Bullying, depression, and suicidal ideation in Finnish adolescents: School survey. *BMJ, 319*(7206), 348–351. https://doi.org/10.1136/bmj.319.7206.348

Kealy, D., Laverdière, O., Cox, D. W., & Hewitt, P. L. (2020). Childhood emotional neglect and depressive and anxiety symptoms among mental health outpatients: The mediating roles of narcissistic vulnerability and shame. *Journal of Mental Health*, 1–9. https://doi.org/10.1080/09638237.2020.1836557

Keeley, B. (2021). *The state of the world's children 2021: On my mind–promoting, protecting and caring for children's mental health* (p. 10017). UNICEF. 3 United Nations Plaza, New York, NY.

Kemp, S. (2022, Feb 16). *Digital 2022: Mongolia.* Digital 2022: Mongolia—DataReportal–Global Digital Insights.

Khantzian, E. J. (1997). The self-medication hypothesis of substance use disorders: A reconsideration and recent applications. *Harvard Review of Psychiatry, 4*(5), 231–244.

Latimer, S., Covic, T., Cumming, S. R., & Tennant, A. (2009). Psychometric analysis of the Self-Harm Inventory using Rasch modelling. *BMC Psychiatry, 9*(1), 1–9. https://doi.org/10.1186/1471-244X-9-53

Lee, T., & Cornell, D. (2009). Concurrent validity of the Olweus bully/victim questionnaire. *Journal of School Violence, 9*(1), 56–73. https://doi.org/10.1080/15388220903185613

Lee, H., Lee, E. Y., Greene, B., & Shin, Y. J. (2019). Psychological distress among adolescents in Laos, Mongolia, Nepal, and Sri Lanka. *Asian Nursing Research, 13*(2), 147–153. https://doi.org/10.1016/j.anr.2019.04.001

Lodi, E., Boerchi, D., Magnano, P., & Patrizi, P. (2019). High-School satisfaction scale (H-Sat Scale): Evaluation of contextual satisfaction in relation to High-School Students' life satisfaction. *Behavioral Sciences, 9*(12), 125. https://doi.org/10.3390/bs9120125

Lui, P. P., & Rollock, D. (2013). Tiger mother: Popular and psychological scientific perspectives on Asian culture and parenting. *American Journal of Orthopsychiatry, 83*(4), 450. https://doi.org/10.1111/ajop.12043

Mehlum, L., Ramleth, R. K., Tørmoen, A. J., Haga, E., Diep, L. M., Stanley, B. H., et al. (2019). Long term effectiveness of dialectical behavior therapy versus enhanced usual care for adolescents with self-harming and suicidal behavior. *Journal of Child Psychology and Psychiatry, 60*(10), 1112–1122. https://doi.org/10.1111/jcpp.13077

Milot Travers, A. S., & Mahalik, J. R. (2021). Positive youth development as a protective factor for adolescents at risk for depression and alcohol use. *Applied Developmental Science, 25*(4), 322–331. https://doi.org/10.1080/10888691.2019.1634569

Monahan, K. C., Oesterle, S., Rhew, I., & Hawkins, J. D. (2014). The relation between risk and protective factors for problem behaviors and depressive symptoms, antisocial behavior, and alcohol use in adolescence. *Journal of Community Psychology, 42*(5), 621–638. https://doi.org/10.1002/jcop.21642

Montgomery, S. C., Donnelly, M., Bhatnagar, P., Carlin, A., Kee, F., & Hunter, R. F. (2020). Peer social network processes and adolescent health behaviors: A systematic review. *Preventive Medicine, 130*, 105900. https://doi.org/10.1016/j.ypmed.2019.105900

Nash, J. K., & Bowen, G. L. (2002). Defining and estimating risk and protection: An illustration from the school success profile. *Child and Adolescent Social Work Journal, 19*(3), 247–261. https://doi.org/10.1023/A:1015532132061

National Statistics' Commission. (2021). *End of the year report for Mongolian population.*

Olson, D. (2011). FACES IV and the circumplex model: Validation study. *Journal of Marital and Family Therapy, 37*(1), 64–80. https://doi.org/10.1111/j.1752-0606.2009.00175.x

Olweus, D. (1996). Revised Olweus bully/victim questionnaire. *Journal of Psychopathology and Behavioral Assessment.*

Papachristou, E., & Flouri, E. (2020). The codevelopment of internalizing symptoms, externalizing symptoms, and cognitive ability across childhood and adolescence. *Development and Psychopathology, 32*(4), 1375–1389. https://doi.org/10.1017/S0954579419001330

Pozzar, R., Hammer, M. J., Underhill-Blazey, M., Wright, A. A., Tulsky, J. A., Hong, F., et al. (2020). Threats of bots and other bad actors to data quality following research participant recruitment through social media: Cross-sectional questionnaire. *Journal of Medical Internet Research, 22*(10), e23021. https://doi.org/10.2196/2302

Rarick, C., Winter, G., Barczyk, C., Pruett, M., & Nickerson, I. (2014). Mongolia: A cultural portrait using the Hofstede 5-D model. *Global Journal of Management and Business Research.*

Sansone, R. A., & Sansone, L. A. (2010). Measuring self-harm behavior with the self-harm inventory. *Psychiatry (edgmont), 7*(4), 16.

Santor, D. A., Messervey, D., & Kusumakar, V. (2000). Measuring peer pressure, popularity, and conformity in young adolescent boys and girls: Predicting school performance, sexual attitudes, and substance use. *Journal of Youth and Adolescence., 29*, 163–218. https://doi.org/10.1023/A:1005152515264

Shi, Q., Ettekal, I., Deutz, M. H., & Woltering, S. (2020). Trajectories of pure and co-occurring internalizing and externalizing problems from early childhood to adolescence: Associations with early childhood individual and contextual antecedents. *Developmental Psychology, 56*(10), 1906. https://doi.org/10.1037/dev0001095

Simantov, E., Schoen, C., & Klein, J. D. (2000). Health-compromising behaviors: Why do adolescents smoke or drink? Identifying underlying risk and protective factors. *Archives of Pediatrics & Adolescent Medicine, 154*(10), 1025–1033. https://doi.org/10.1001/archpedi.154.10.1025

Sodnom, O. (2020). *Risk factors associated with adolescents smoking in Mongolia* (Doctoral dissertation, Graduate School of Public Health).

Steinhausen, H. C., & Metzke, C. W. (1998). Youth self-report of behavioral and emotional problems in a Swiss epidemiological study. *Journal of Youth and Adolescence, 27*(4), 429–441. https://doi.org/10.1023/A:1022895917868

Straus, M. A., Kinard, E., & Williams, L. M. (1997). The neglect scale.

Streiner, D. L. (2003). Starting at the beginning: An introduction to coefficient alpha and internal consistency. *Journal of Personality Assessment, 80*(1), 99–103. https://doi.org/10.1207/S15327752JPA8001_18

Talevi, D., Socci, V., Carai, M., Carnaghi, G., Faleri, S., Trebbi, E., et al. (2020). Mental health outcomes of the CoViD-19 pandemic. *Rivista di psichiatria, 55*(3), 137–144.

Tiesel, J., & Olson, D. H. (1997). FACES IV: Reliability and validity. *Unpublished manuscript, University of Minnesota.*

Tillmann, S., Tobin, D., Avison, W., & Gilliland, J. (2018). Mental health benefits of interactions with nature in children and teenagers: A systematic review. *Journal of Epidemiology and Community Health, 72*(10), 958–966.

Uba, I., Yaacob, S. N., Juhari, R., & Talib, M. A. (2010). Effect of self-esteem on the relationship between depression and bullying among teenagers in Malaysia. *Asian Social Science, 6*(12), 77–85.

Vanchindorj, B., Bayartsogt, B., Yerlan, G., Narm, A., Naidansuren, T., Batdelger, S., et al. (2017). Prevalence of emotional and behavioral problems among adolescence and some risk factors in Mongolia. *Asean Journal of Psychiatry, 18*(2), 1–14.

Veiga, F., & Leite, A. (2016). Adolescents' self-concept short scale: A version of PHCSCS. *Procedia Social and Behavioral Sciences, 217*, 631–637. https://doi.org/10.1016/j.sbspro.2016.02.079

Warschburger, P., & Zitzmann, J. (2018). The efficacy of a universal school-based prevention program for eating disorders among German adolescents: Results from a randomized-controlled trial. *Journal of Youth and Adolescence, 47*(6), 1317–1331. https://doi.org/10.1007/s10964-018-0852-3

Windle, M. (2003). Alcohol use among adolescents and young adults. *Alcohol Research & Health, 27*(1), 79.

World Health Organization. (2001). *The second decade: Improving adolescent health and development* (No. WHO/FRH/ADH/98.18 Rev. 1). World Health Organization.

Yang, B., Xiong, C., & Huang, J. (2021). Parental emotional neglect and left-behind children's externalizing problem behaviors: The mediating role of deviant peer affiliation and the moderating role of beliefs about adversity. *Children and Youth Services Review, 120*, 105710. https://doi.org/10.1016/j.childyouth.2020.105710

Young, K. A. (2020). Exploring the psychometric properties of two primary domains in the Revised Olweus Bully/Victim Questionnaire (R-OBVQ) among primary school learners in South Africa. *Journal of Psychopathology and Behavioral Assessment, 42*(3), 539–545. https://doi.org/10.1007/s10862-020-09787-7

The Effect of Manipulations and Time on Episodic Memory: Investigation with Movies

Yunke Chen

Abstract Based on the dissociation observed between episodic and semantic memory, the determinants of episodic memory recall have been investigated via various approaches. The present study is based on the experiment data of (Tang et al., Scientific Reports 6:1–14, 2016) evaluating participants' performance in recognizing movie frames. Their experiment measured the recognition accuracy of 161 participants in total, with frames of two episodes from the TV series "24", Season 6. Compared to adopting individual words or images as stimuli, the approach to investigate episodic memory with movie frames involves temporal and spatial contextual information into the memory process, which signifies some key features of real-life episodic narrative beyond semantic memory. It is also more controllable than the neuropsychological method which observes the autobiographical memories of amnesic patients. The present study conducted Bayesian ANOVA and *t* tests to compare the performance when the movie frames had different variables manipulated. It replicated the previous finding that the manipulations of sound removal, temporal reversal, 75% area occlusion, and motion removal significantly affect people's recognizing performance for a movie frame, suggesting these features as influential for episodic memory. There was no significant difference in performance with different retention times between studying and testing, so the result does not indicate a significant effect of time on memory recall. The findings on the determinants of episodic memory recalling performance may cater to the need of enhancing episodic memory performance in applications like collecting testimony from eyewitnesses and memorization tasks involving episodic narratives.

Keywords Episodic memory · Recognition memory · Memory retention

Y. Chen (✉)
Department of Psychology, The University of Hong Kong, Hong Kong, China
e-mail: cyk1028@connect.hku.hk

P. Macaulay and L. Tan (eds.), *Applied Psychology Readings*,
https://doi.org/10.1007/978-981-99-2613-8_2

1 Introduction

In the study of explicit memory, episodic memory refers to the system of localizing events in specific time epochs. In comparison to semantic memory, which is knowledge not tied to one's experience of time, it could mean "remembering" beyond merely "knowing" (Tulving, 1985). A double dissociation observed between episodic and semantic memory cases support the specialty of episodic memory, which has been evidenced widely in both clinical cases (De Renzi et al., 1987; Kitchener et al., 1998; Rosenbaum et al., 2005) and brain-imaging studies, including positron emission tomography (PET) and functional magnetic resonance imaging (FMRI) (Buckner et al., 2000; Tulving, 2002).

Based on the idea that episodic memory carries narratives of autonoetic experiences, there is a gap between all the information input and what is encoded in episodic narratives (Tulving, 2002). Concerning the gap, plentiful literature has investigated the determinants of whether one kind of external information can be encoded in and recalled from episodic memory. Multiple variables about the content that is memorized probably contribute to varied levels of episodic memory recollection (Vogt & Magnussen, 2007). There has also been rich evidence for the intuitive idea that memory fades with time, such as examinations of the forgetfulness of regularity over time ever since Ebbinghaus (1885) modeled his classic forgetting curve (Andermane & Bowers, 2015; Furman et al., 2007; Hu et al., 2013; Murre & Dros, 2015). Some features of participants like gender and age have been investigated as well (Grysman, 2017). Previously adopted methods to examine these variables range from tests with static images, separate words, sequential visual narratives, to transcranial magnetic stimulation (TMS) and the neuropsychological observations of clinical cases (Bayley et al., 2003; Hebscher & Voss, 2020; Magliano et al., 2017; Rosenbaum et al., 2008; Tang et al., 2016).

The present study is based on a previous study by Tang et al. (2016) named "Predicting episodic memory formation for movie events". Their experiment investigated the relationship between near-real-life scenarios and episodic memory performance by evaluating participants' performance of recognizing movie frames with different manipulated variables. They manipulated variables about the memorized content and the retention time between encoding and testing. The memory material adopted for this purpose are movie frames with multiple variables manipulated, such as with sound removed, temporal sequence reversed, or adapted into static frames. Their findings classified sound removal, temporal order reversal, and occlusion of 75% image area as manipulations that cause significant decrease in memory performance, so they are labeled "high-level manipulations". The horizontal flipping of the frames and color removal led to no significant difference in performance and were categorized as two "low-level manipulations". They also attempted to model episodic memory formation dependent on these evaluated variables.

Based on data collected in their experiment, the present study aims at replicating the previous result about the manipulations' effect on recalling performance and further investigating the effect of time. First, as the previous result was analyzed with a two-sided non-parametric permutation test, we seek to obtain more solid evidence for the findings. Thus, we replicate the data analysis with Bayes Factor *t* test and ANOVA, and add an additional variable of motion, which was not analyzed in the previous research. We hypothesize that similar effects on the memory performance will be observed with each manipulation, and the additional manipulation of motion will cause significant effect, too. Second, the present research differs from the previous study in investigating the effect of retention time. Although Tang et al. (2016) collected experimental data from varied retention time, they did not analyze the effect of time across testing sessions. Nor have the existing research on the effect of time examined the interaction effect between time and the material manipulations on the episodic memory performance (Andermane & Bowers, 2015; Furman et al., 2007). Therefore, the present study examined the performance difference across varied retention time in each manipulated condition and their interaction effect with each manipulation. Given the previous literature supporting the memory decrease with time, it is hypothesized that we will observe worse performance in later time sessions than earlier ones (Andermane & Bowers, 2015; Furman et al., 2007; Hu et al., 2013; Murre & Dros, 2015).

2 Methods

2.1 Experiment Procedure: The Original Study

The original experiment by Tang et al. (2016) included 161 participants in total. The material adopted as the near-real-life movie stimuli was Episode 1 and Episode 2 from Season 6 of the TV series "24". In their experiment, no participants had watched any episode prior to the encoding stage.

All participants went through an experiment procedure designed as described below: in the encoding stage, the participants watched a clip of the chosen movie. After a period of retention, they were tested on their performance in recalling the movie content. They were shown movie frames that are either studied frames that they had studied in the encoding stage or foil frames that are new to them. The frames were presented in pseudo-random order, and on each frame, participants were asked to determine whether it was frames that they were previously exposed to or new, foil frames. The number of studied frames and foil frames presented were equal, so they were equal in the probability of appearance, and the performance at chance level was 50%.

The original study conducted four experiments in total. First, to examine the validity of the experiment design, there was a main experiment testing the general level of memorability for the stimuli, which were shots and frames in movies in their design. This experiment showed a high rate of memorization for the stimuli even though the targets and foils were similar frames from two sequential episodes, Episode 1 and Episode 2, respectively. It supported the argument that the participants had memory performance above chance and below ceiling, leaving an ample range to investigate which variables contribute to varied levels of memory performance. Then, two variant experiments, Variant 1 and Variant 2 were carried out to test the generalizability of the conclusions from the main experiment. As the main experiment adopted frames from Episode 1 of the movie as the material for studied frames and Episode 2 as the material for foil frames, Variant 1 focusing on the effect of the difference among episodes. It switched the application of Episode 1 and Episode 2 and successfully replicated the findings in the main experiment, finding little influence from the variation in episodes. Variant 2 targeted the interference from the repetitive testing that each participant experience in multiple sessions. Although the test frames that appeared in the 6 test sessions are different, the same subjects went through repeated tests with frames from the same movie episode. As repeated exposure may lead to better performance in later sessions and act as a confound in the experiment, Variant 2 tested each subject only in one session. They found a small but significant result of lower performance than the former two experiments (79.2 $\pm$ 5.9% cf. 85.6 $\pm$ 5.3% in the main experiment). However, it is still consistent to the qualitative conclusions in the previous experiments: even in Variant 2, the performance remains higher than chance level (50%) and lower than ceiling level. Hence, they decided not to alter the experiment design and proceeded to Variant 3 to assess the effect of manipulations.

Based on these three tests, Variant 3 was conducted to test all the manipulated features of the memory stimuli. The manipulations they made to the movie stimuli include (1) removing the sound; (2) presenting static, single frames instead of video shots with motion; (3) flipping the frames horizontally; (4) replacing the color with grayscale shades; (5) reversing the temporal sequence that frames appear; and (6) occluding three randomly selected quadrant of the frame. They recorded the participants' performance in the new/old determining test across six sequential sessions, each with increasing retention time since the encoding stage. The six sessions range from right after the encoding to around 24 h, 7 days, 30 days, 90 days, and one year later. Each subject participated in different number of sessions. Experimenters obtained the percentage of correct responses from 52 subjects in each combination of manipulation and session. The present study analyzes the data collected in this experiment.

2.2 *Data Analysis: The Present Study*

The data from experiment Variant 3 by Tang et al. (2016) were from 52 subjects and six sessions. Among them, we removed the data from six subjects who participated in two or less sessions. Only eight subjects participated in Session 6, and it is few compared to 16 participants in Session 5 and more of them in even earlier sessions. For the sake of larger subject size for the comparison across time sessions, the observations from Session 6 are not included in the analysis either. After these removals, the present analysis is based on a total of 165,860 responses from 46 subjects across five sessions. The later one session is, the longer is the corresponding retention time between encoding and testing. When a session is later, there is longer retention time between encoding and testing. We divided the number of correct answers with the total number of tests to obtain the accuracy of participants' performance in each condition, testing six kinds of manipulations: sound removal, static frames, horizontal flipping, color removal, temporal reversal, and occlusion of random three-quarters of the image. Then, we analyzed the data with a Bayes Factor *t* test and a Bayes Factor analysis of variance (ANOVA) using R studio (Morey & Rouder, 2015; R Core Team, 2020).

First, we attempted to replicate the original study with Bayes Factor *t* tests. We compared the participants' recognition accuracy between manipulated and not manipulated conditions, such as with or without sound, to examine the null hypotheses that the participants' accuracies are the same between manipulated and not manipulated conditions. If the null hypotheses are rejected, the alternative hypotheses would be that there are significant effects of the manipulations on the participants' episodic memory recalling performance.

Secondly, to test the effect of time in relation to different manipulations, we adopted the Bayes Factor ANOVA to compare the accuracy across five sessions, with different conditions combined. The data were examined against the null hypothesis that participants' accuracies in the tests are the same in the five sessions. The alternative hypothesis would be that their accuracies are not the same over time, suggesting a significant effect of time on their memory performance. In addition to overall effect of the variable time, we tested the interaction effect between time and each variable with Bayes Factor ANOVA. We compared the accuracy across sessions in each 12 conditions (with/without manipulation * six types of conditions). We examined the data against the null hypothesis that in each condition, participants' accuracies are the same across time sessions. If the null hypothesis were rejected, we would embrace the alternative hypothesis that the element of retention time has a significant interaction effect on the influence of the material-related variables.

3 Result

In the six Bayes Factor *t* tests on the six types of manipulations, the null hypothesis (H_0) is that there is no difference in recognition accuracy between the manipulated and not manipulated conditions for each manipulation. For the manipulation of sound removal, the Bayes factor indicates evidence for H_+. As is shown in Table 1, BF_{+0} = 4.27E+23, meaning that the response data are approximately 34.6 times more likely to occur under the circumstance of H_+ rather than H_0. It indicates strong evidence in favor of H_+. The result is similar for the variables of motion (BF_{+0} = 2.64E+44), temporal reversal (BF_{+0} = 6.19E+17) and 75% image occlusion (BF_{+0} = 7.69E+48). The tests all provide strong evidence for H_+, which is that these manipulations have significant effects on the participants' accuracy in the recognizing test. According to the *t* test on the manipulation of horizontal flipping, BF_{+0} = 6.53, meaning that it

Table 1 Bayes Factor *t* test and ANOVA

Experience condition	Bayes factor *t* test	Bayes factor ANOVA
Sound_on	4.26564E+23	0.42
Sound_off		0.082
Static_on	2.64477E+44	0.07
Static_off		0.193
Flip_on	6.525067	0.044
Flip_off		0.374
Gray_on	0.09406201	0.215
Gray_off		0.28
Reverse_on	6.1902E+17	0.445
Reverse_off		0.604
Occlude_on	7.68592E+48	370,393.2
Occlude_off		1.923

is approximately 6.5 times more likely to obtain the data under H_+ than under H_0. This result indicates moderate evidence for H_+. The tests on color removal indicate strong evidence in favor of H_0: $BF_{+0} = 0.09$, which means that the data are about 11.1 times more likely to occur in the condition of H_0 compared to H_+.

In the Bayes Factor ANOVA tests comparing the recognition accuracies across the five testing sessions, the null hypothesis (H_0) is that the recognition accuracy is the same across all the time sessions. As illustrated in Fig. 1, this test indicates no evidence for H_+. Specifically, $BF_{+0} = 0.08$, which means that the data are approximately 12.5 times more likely to occur under H_0 than under H_+, so it indicates strong evidence for H_0.

As for the Bayesian ANOVA on the interaction effect between time and the 12 manipulation conditions, the null hypothesis (H_0) is that in each condition, the recognition accuracy is the same across all time sessions. As displayed in Fig. 3, tests in most of the 12 conditions indicates no evidence for H_+, except the condition with the manipulation of 75% frames area occlusion. In particular, without the manipulation of sound removal (as in "sound_on"), $BF_{+0} = 0.42$, meaning that it is approximately 2.4 times more likely to obtain the data under H_0, so it indicates anecdotal evidence in favor of H_0. With the sound-removal manipulation (as in "sound_off"), $BF_{+0} = 0.08$, meaning that the data are around 12.5 times more likely to occur with H_0, indicating strong evidence for H_0. Similarly, with respect to the manipulation of motion removal, the tests indicate strong evidence for H_0 with the manipulation as in "static_on" ($BF_{+0} = 0.07$) and moderate evidence for H_0 without the manipulation as in "static_off" ($BF_{+0} = 0.19$). The tests for the manipulation of horizontal flipping showed strong evidence for H_0 ($BF = 0.04$) with this manipulation as in "flip_on". Without this manipulation, there is also anecdotal evidence for H_0 ($BF_{+0} = 0.37$) as in "flip_off". There is moderate evidence for H_0 with the manipulation of color removal as in "color_on" ($BF_{+0} = 0.22$) or without this manipulation as in "color_

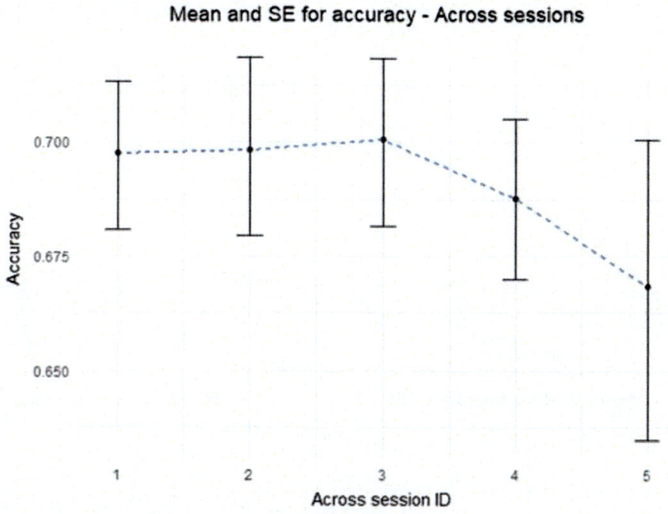

Fig. 1 The recognition accuracy across each time session

off" (BF_{+0} = 0.28). There is anecdotal evidence for H_0 with the manipulation of temporal reversal, without this manipulation, or without the manipulation of 75% area occlusion ("reverse_on": BF_{+0} = 0.45; "reverse_off": BF_{+0} = 0.6; "occlude_off": BF_{+0} = 1.92). However, in the condition with the manipulation of 75% occlusion (as in "occlude_on"), BF_{+0} = 370,393.2, meaning that the data is over 370,000 times more likely to occur under H_+ than H_0, indicating strong evidence for H_+.

According to a post-hoc Tukey Test comparing the recognition accuracies among the five sessions in the "occlude_on" condition, the accuracy in Session 3 is significantly higher than that in the other four sessions ($p < 0.001$), while there was no significant difference between other pairs of sessions ($p > 0.5$) (see Figs. 2, 3, and 4).

4 Discussion

Regarding the six manipulations to movie content, our test results are supportive of the effects of the features of sound, motion, sequence reversal, and occlusion on the performance of episodic memory reflected in recognition tests. Meanwhile, the result provides evidence in favor of the effect of horizontal flipping, but the evidence is weaker. The result indicates no effect from color removal on episodic memory performance. The replication attempt validates the significant effect on memory performance of the elements rated as "high-level manipulations" in the original study, adding to it the manipulation of motion removal (Tang et al., 2016). Our analyses also support the finding that the effect of the two "low-level manipulations" were less prominent than the other elements regarding their interference with episodic

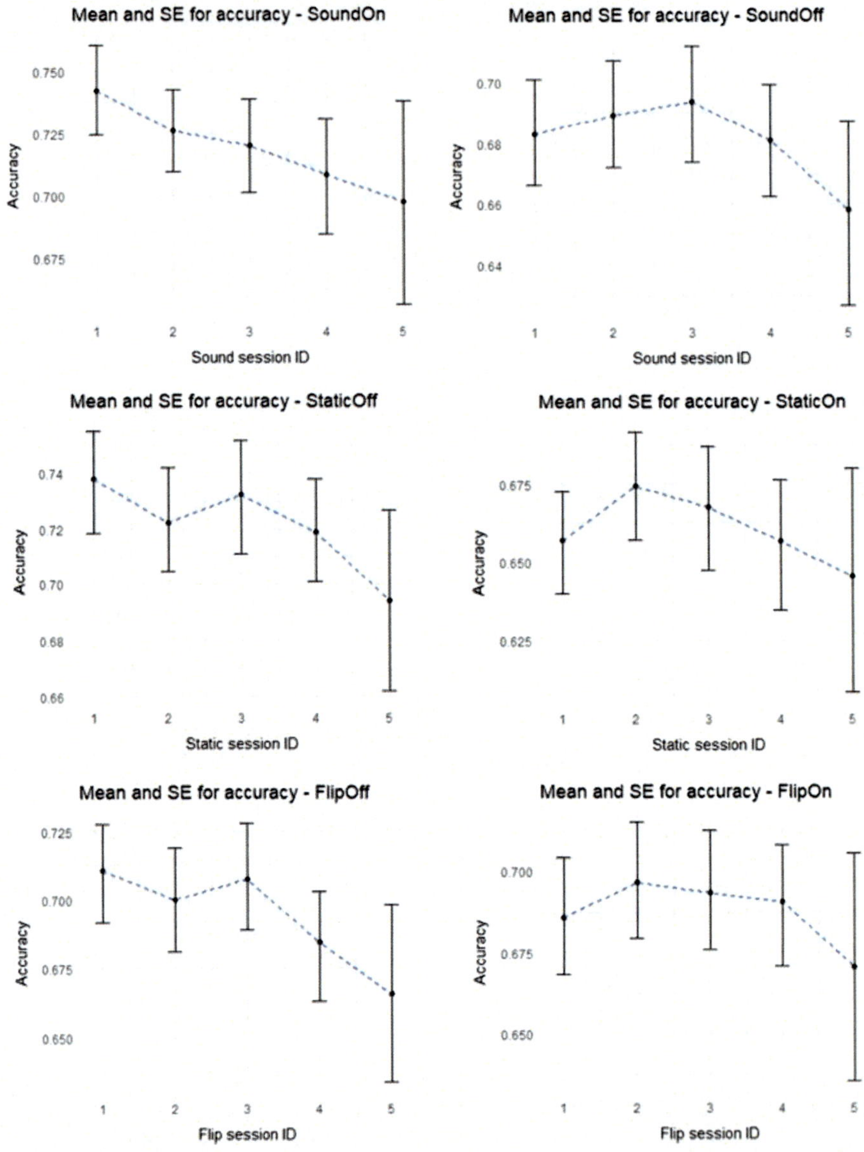

Fig. 2 The recognition accuracy across each time session in each manipulation condition

memory formation and recollection. Hence, the present result is consistent with the original study, and the evaluation of the manipulations to the memory materials was successfully replicated.

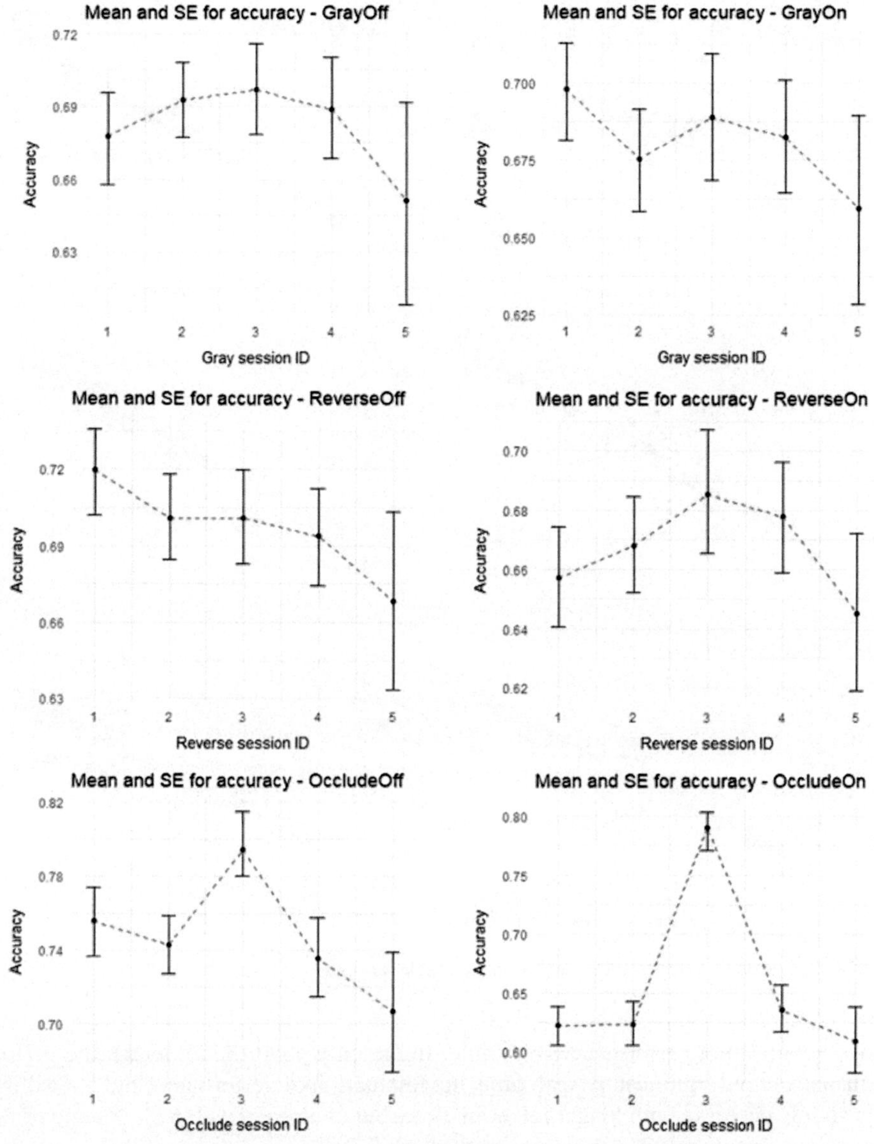

Fig. 2 (continued)

Concerning the effect of time, the present study found no evidence for a change in episodic memory performance over varied retention time. As for the interaction effect between time and manipulations, the results indicate no evidence for varied performance across time in most conditions except for the condition with the occlusion manipulation. In this condition, the third session showed prominently better performance than the other sessions. Nonetheless, the results provided no evidence

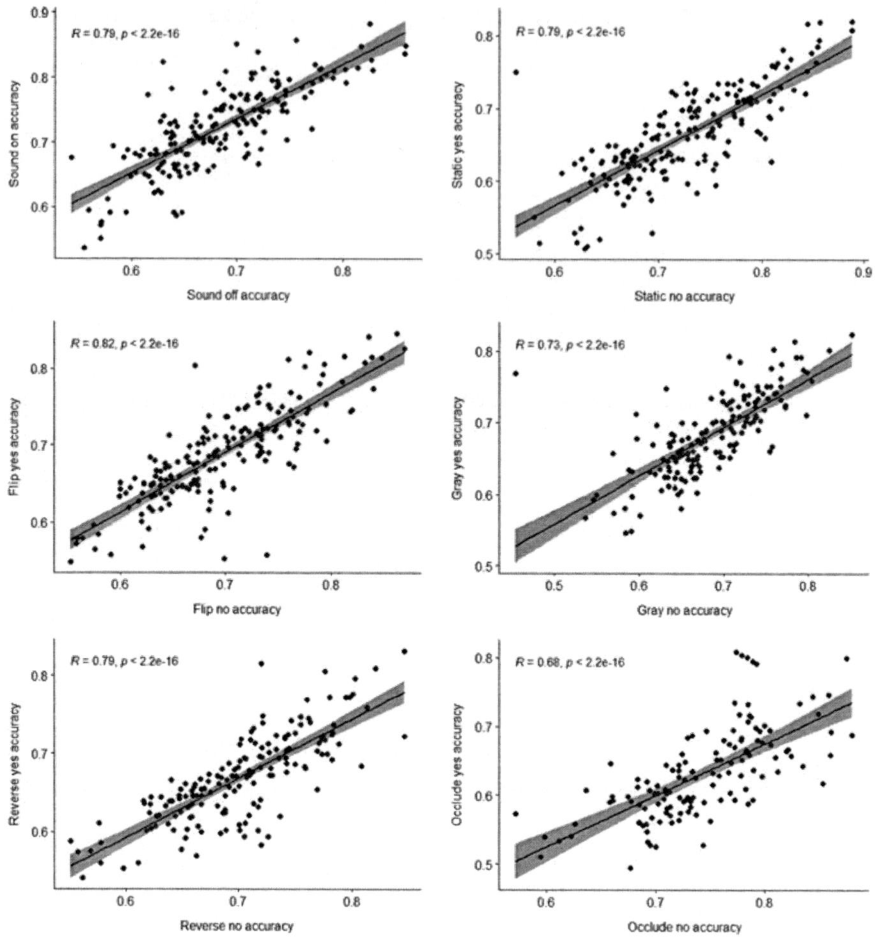

Fig. 3 Correlation between manipulations for each variable

for a worsening performance over time: in the only condition in which the performance altered significantly with time, the fluctuation of performance did not exhibit a simple decrease with longer retention time, but one peak level in the middle of the sessions. In other words, there was an increase followed by a decrease. Moreover, the level of performance in the last session was not significantly different from the level in the earliest two sessions. Therefore, the results indicate no significant decrease across time sessions, against our hypothesis based on memory's fading with time.

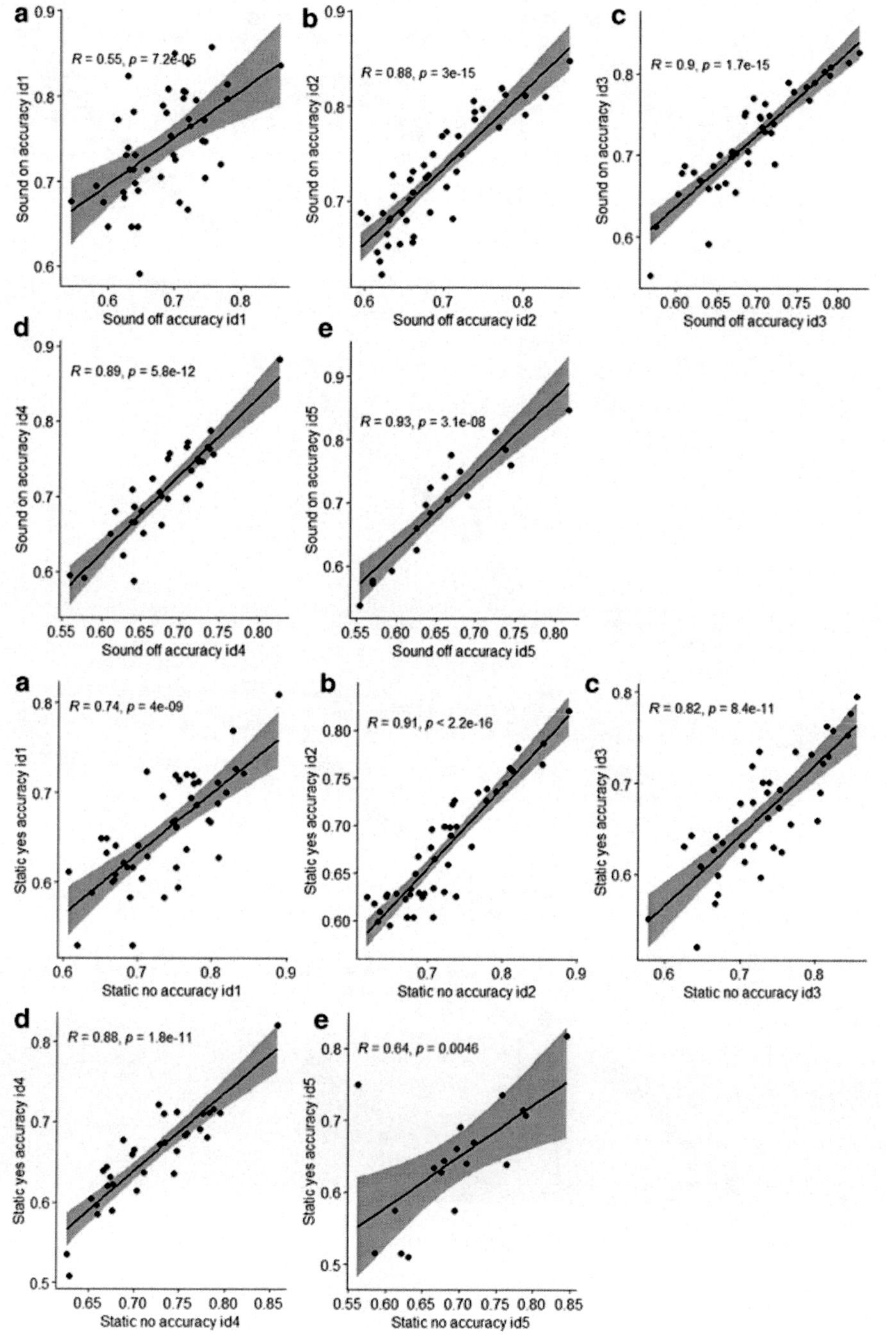

Fig. 4 Correlation between manipulations for each variable in each session

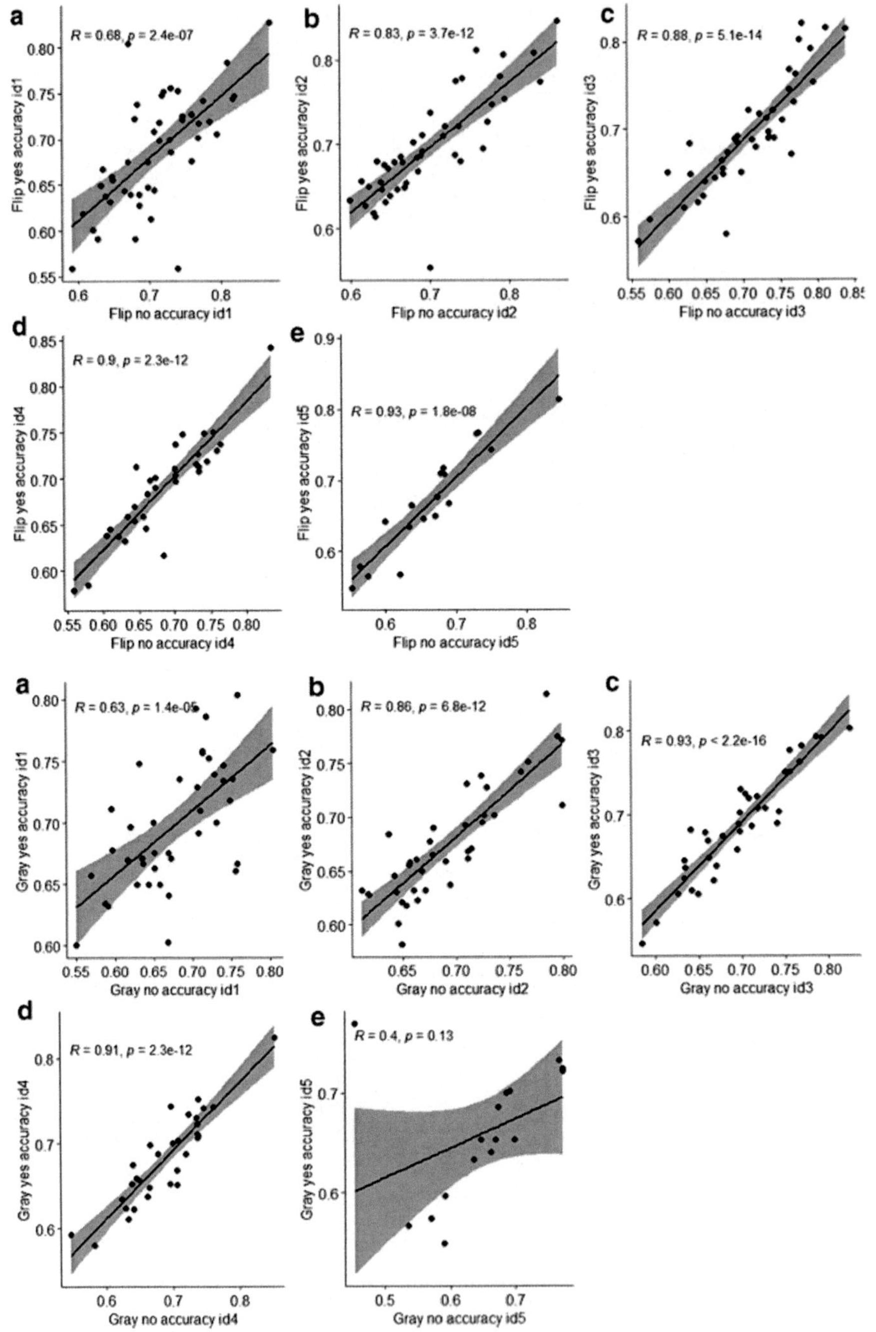

Fig. 4 (continued)

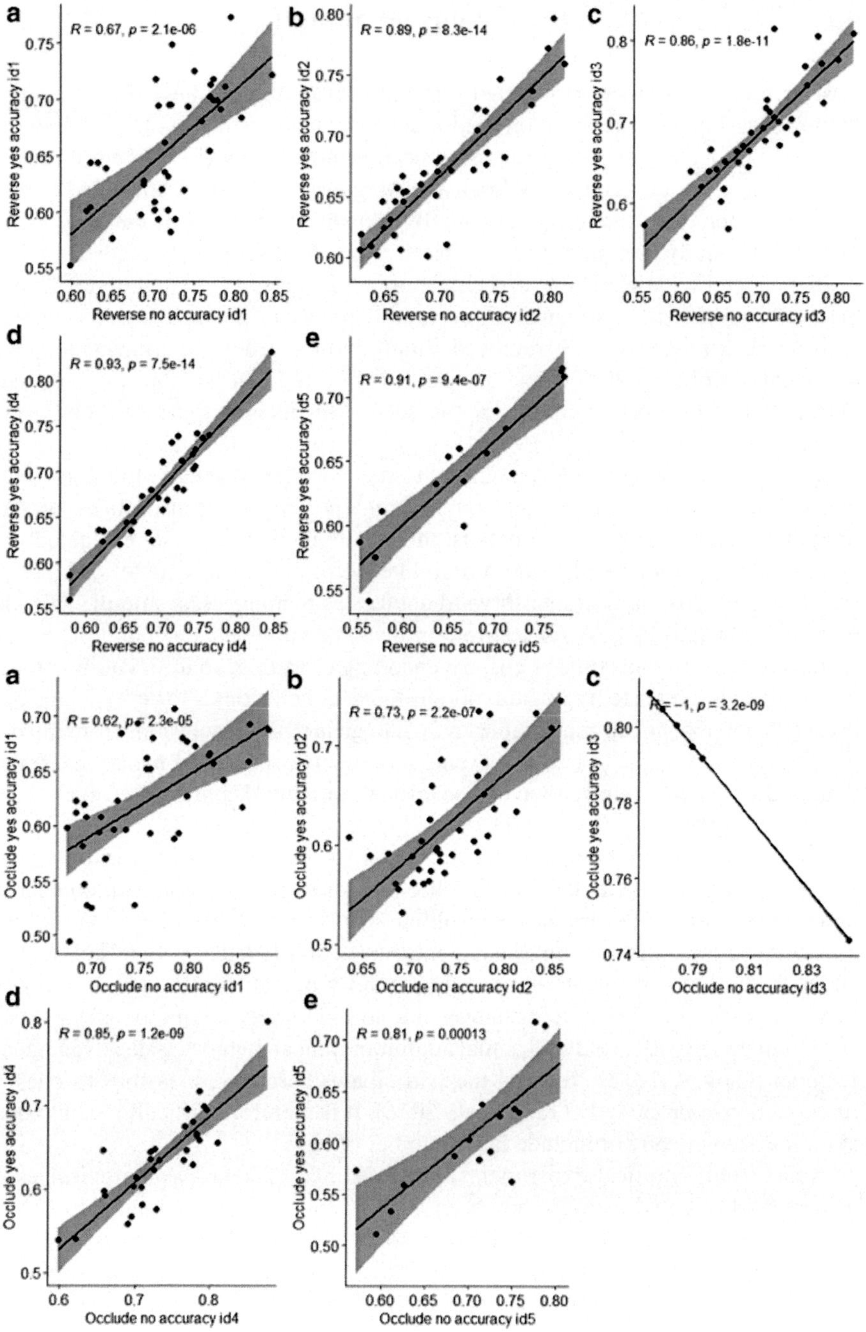

Fig. 4 (continued)

4.1 The Effect of Manipulations on Stimuli

Based on the experiment conducted through movie stimuli, these findings add to the growing body of literature on the influence of features of memorized materials on episodic memory encoding that have been acquired through different measures. For instance, the experiment of Vogt and Magnussen (2007) exemplified another feature of memory content that potentially influences the level of memory formation. In this study, researchers asked participants to discriminate studied pictures from distractors that were new to them, adopting images of different doors. Experimenters compared the distinguishing accuracy between original pictures and pictures with some extraneous details removed, and found the group experimented without the detail performing 20% worse. Hence, it is inferred that the object details facilitate pictorial memory encoding of the scenes by including richer recognizable information.

Vogt and Magnussen (2007) managed to select images that carry the same motif, doors, thus controlling the variable of image content. They could also edit the pictures to include or exclude irrelevant details, thus manipulating the exact evaluated variables artificially. Individual, static stimuli like words and images of faces, objects, or scenes are effective and straightforward choices as memory tests stimuli. This kind of stimuli is relatively easy for controlling involved variables. Each unit of material requires relatively short time or cost for encoding or testing, so the recalling process can be operated repeatedly to gain more reliable conclusions. However, it has been argued that it may not be convincible enough to generalize conclusions from separate words or static images to real-life events that involve sequential narratives, for the temporal and spatial information can be critical for natural context (Lee et al., 2020; Tang et al., 2016).

On the other hand, compared to individual stimuli in laboratory setting, inferring knowledge from the recall of real-life memories features a natural context but more challenges to the variables controlling. Multiple studies focusing on the autobiographical memories of amnesic patients have contributed to people's knowledge about the brain areas related to episodic memory operations (Bayley et al., 2003; Rosenbaum et al., 2008). Nevertheless, due to the variety among people's experience in their daily life, studying actual autobiographical memory is disadvantageous for controlling variables, such as the participants' practice, exposure to cues, or reproduction appropriately (Tang et al., 2016). It is therefore difficult to study these stimuli systematically or include large number of tests.

Apart from empirical experiments and reference of neuropsychological cases, a more sophisticated measure has been transcranial magnetic stimulation (TMS), meaning stimulating neurons in different areas of the cerebral cortex with electric currents and observing the affected brain functions. It has been a recent argument for the possibility to examine understandings of episodic memory network via TMS non-invasively (Hebscher & Voss, 2020). Nevertheless, there may still be some time before this technology can be applied to episodic memory widely (Pascual-Leone et al., 2000).

Synthesizing the above-mentioned characteristics, an alternative approach that balances the representativeness of natural situations and the feasibility for manipulation and repetitive application would be preferable for investigating episodic memory properties in empirical experiments. Hence, we propose movie as an accessible and effective source of material. Researchers can obtain narrative memory materials from movies, ranging from audiovisual clips of videos to sequential frames and story plots.

The history of applying moving images to investigate memory recall can be traced back to existing literature by Boring (1916), who suggested that witnessing criminal events is like encoding movies into memory. Thus, by testing the witnesses' capacity to report moving pictures, people can infer the reliability of their crime report.

Although the approach that adopts repetition of randomized, separate stimuli has prevailed among the episodic memory studies in a long period of time, recently, the utility of images containing narratives has been reported to increase (Lee et al., 2020; Magliano et al., 2017). For instance, an experiment asked participants to fill in gaps among sequential narrative images to explore implications of memory recalling and inferential processing (Magliano et al., 2017). Compared to individual words or images, they feature information about the temporal sequence, spatial environment, engaging plots, emotions, and so on (Tang et al., 2016). Apart from the "ecological validity" as Lee et al., (2020, p. 111) summarized, arguably, narratives stimulate brain structures and processes beyond what content without narratives stimulates. For instance, as for sequential images, a recent paper indicated a complexity in the bidirectional information transition between visual narratives and episodic memory (Cohn, 2020). Accordingly, despite the ubiquity of visual narrative usage, such as in instruction pictures and comic strips for children, their creation and understanding requires a proficiency that is obtained through complicated learning and brain functions. Hence, it is believed that movie cuts, a form of narrative containing both visual and auditory information, can be a kind of material that both simulate real-life events and provide convenience for variable controlling.

4.2 *The Effect of Time Sessions*

As for the second part, the results from the present study are unsupportive of the hypothesis that episodic memory performance worsens with longer time after encoding. Much previous empirical evidence has been in favor of this hypothesis, including those adopting similar stimuli, movies, or different material as memory content. For an example involving similar choice of stimuli, Furman et al. (2007) asked participants to watch a 27 min' long movie and tested their performance in recall and recognition tasks and their metamemory confidence about events in the movie. They compared the test responses after a delay time ranging from three hours to nine months, and the results indicated worse performance corresponding to longer delay (Furman et al., 2007). As for experiments adopting different materials, the study of Andermane and Bowers (2015) compared participants' accuracy in distinguishing studied images of static objects from foil images after one week's retention time with their performance right after studying the images. Adopting thousands of images of different objects, they found a significant reduction in visual long-term memory recalling following the week's retention, thus verifying the hypothesis. In comparison to them, the present analysis failed to obtain evidence for the memory decrease with time.

One probable contributor to this result lies in the methodological limitation of repetitive exposure. As has been explained in the methodology, the participants were repeatedly exposed to testing stimuli, which are movie frames from the same two episodes. Even if no frame has been presented to them more than once, and no feedback has been provided to them following any response, they may obtain cues from the events in the movie plot, other features of the narratives, or be more proficient in making similar judgments over repeated test sessions. They were likely to perform better over time due to the repetition alone, thus counteracting the effect of time that worsen the performance over time. The experiment Variant 2 has verified a small but significant effect of the repetitive exposure with the result of lower performance following an experiment design that tests each participant in only one session compared to the design with repetitive testing. Although the performance level with this limitation is still valid for examining the manipulated variables of the material, it may cause a quantitative difference that interferes with the investigation on the effect of retention time. Therefore, to obtain more valid measurements of the effect of time, a follow-up study could be conducted adopting the alternative experiment design in Variant 2 to eliminate the interference of repetitive exposure to the stimuli.

It is acknowledged that apart from the variables of material manipulation and retention time examined at present, another group of elements considered to vary the episodic memory recalling is the features inherent in the tested subjects. This type of factors includes the gender, age, cognitive abilities, and the participants' knowledge prior to the concerned memory encoding. For instance, the experiment by Grysman (2017) exemplifies the difference in gender. His investigation indicates that female performs better than male in recalling autobiographical information details. It specified that females' advantage lies at an early stage after encoding. After that period, the rates of memory decrease do not differ between females and males. Therefore, it is another limitation of the present study to not evaluate the effect of these potential confounders on the episodic memory performance.

5 Conclusion

Based on the response data collected from their experiment, the present study aimed at replicating the previous result about the manipulations' effect on recalling performance and further investigating the element of time. First, as the previous result was analyzed with a two-sided non-parametric permutation test, we replicated the previous experiment with Bayes Factor *t* test and ANOVA, and added one variable, static or motion, which was not analyzed in the previous research. The variable evaluation of the original experiment was successfully replicated, indicating the significant effect of sound, reversal, occlusion, and the additional manipulation, motion. Second, the present research purpose differs from the previous study in the investigation of the effect of the retention time. Although Tang et al. (2016) collected experiment data from varied retention time, they did not analyze the effect of time (Andermane & Bowers, 2015; Furman et al., 2007). Therefore, the present study examined the performance difference across varied retention time in each manipulated condition, and the interaction effect. It indicated the effect of time not as significant as former research did.

References

Andermane, N., & Bowers, J. S. (2015). Detailed and gist-like visual memories are forgotten at similar rates over the course of a week. *Psychonomic Bulletin & Review, 22*(5), 1358–1363. https://doi.org/10.3758/s13423-015-0800-0

Bayley, P. J., Hopkins, R. O., & Squire, L. R. (2003). Successful recollection of remote autobiographical memories by amnesic patients with medial temporal lobe lesions. *Neuron, 38*(1), 135–144. https://doi.org/10.1016/S0896-6273(03)00156-9

Boring, E. G. (1916). Capacity to report upon moving pictures as conditioned by sex and age. A contribution to the Psychology of Testimony. *Journal of the American Institute of Criminal Law and Criminology, 6*(6), 820–834. https://doi.org/10.2307/1133108

Buckner, R. L., Logan, J., Donaldson, D. I., & Wheeler, M. E. (2000). Cognitive neuroscience of episodic memory encoding. *Acta Psychologica, 105*(2–3), 127–139. https://doi.org/10.1016/S0001-6918(00)00057-3

Cohn, N. (2020). Visual narrative comprehension: Universal or not? *Psychonomic Bulletin & Review, 27*(2), 266–285. https://doi.org/10.3758/s13423-019-01670-1

De Renzi, E., Liotti, M., & Nichelli, P. (1987). Semantic amnesia with preservation of autobiographic memory. A case report. *Cortex, 23*(4), 575–597. https://doi.org/10.1016/S0010-9452(87)80050-3

Ebbinghaus, H. (1885). Forgetting curve. *Memory A Contribution to Experimental Psychology*. Downloaded from http://encarta.msn.com/media,461547609,76157803-1

Furman, O., Dorfman, N., Hasson, U., Davachi, L., & Dudai, Y. (2007). They saw a movie: Long-term memory for an extended audiovisual narrative. *Learning & Memory, 14*(6), 457–467. https://doi.org/10.1101/lm.550407

Grysman, A. (2017). Gender differences in episodic encoding of autobiographical memory. *Journal of Applied Research in Memory and Cognition, 6*(1), 51–59. https://doi.org/10.1016/j.jarmac.2016.07.012

Hebscher, M., & Voss, J. L. (2020). Testing network properties of episodic memory using non-invasive brain stimulation. *Current Opinion in Behavioral Sciences, 32*, 35–42. https://doi.org/10.1016/j.cobeha.2020.01.012

Hu, S. G., Liu, Y., Chen, T. P., Liu, Z., Yu, Q., Deng, L. J., et al. (2013). Emulating the Ebbinghaus forgetting curve of the human brain with a NiO-based memristor. *Applied Physics Letters, 103*(13), 133701. https://doi.org/10.1063/1.4822124

Kitchener, E. G., Hodges, J. R., & McCarthy, R. (1998). Acquisition of post-morbid vocabulary and semantic facts in the absence of episodic memory. *Brain: A Journal of Neurology, 121*(7), 1313–1327. https://doi.org/10.1093/brain/121.7.1313

Lee, H., Bellana, B., & Chen, J. (2020). What can narratives tell us about the neural bases of human memory? *Current Opinion in Behavioral Sciences, 32*, 111–119. https://doi.org/10.1016/j.cobeha.2020.02.007

Magliano, J. P., Kopp, K., Higgs, K., & Rapp, D. N. (2017). Filling in the gaps: Memory implications for inferring missing content in graphic narratives. *Discourse Processes, 54*(8), 569–582. https://doi.org/10.1080/0163853X.2015.1136870

Morey, R. D., & Rouder, J. N. (2015). BayesFactor 0.9.11–1. *Comprehensive R Archive Network.* http://cran.r-project.org/web/packages/BayesFactor/index.html

Murre, J. M., & Dros, J. (2015). Replication and analysis of Ebbinghaus' forgetting curve. *PLoS ONE, 10*(7), e0120644. https://doi.org/10.1371/journal.pone.0120644

Pascual-Leone, A., Walsh, V., & Rothwell, J. (2000). Transcranial magnetic stimulation in cognitive neuroscience-virtual lesion, chronometry, and functional connectivity. *Current Opinion in Neurobiology, 10*(2), 232–237. https://doi.org/10.1016/S0959-4388(00)00081-7

Rosenbaum, R. S., Köhler, S., Schacter, D. L., Moscovitch, M., Westmacott, R., Black, S. E., et al. (2005). The case of KC: Contributions of a memory-impaired person to memory theory. *Neuropsychologia, 43*(7), 989–1021. https://doi.org/10.1016/j.neuropsychologia.2004.10.007

Rosenbaum, R. S., Moscovitch, M., Foster, J. K., Schnyer, D. M., Gao, F., Kovacevic, N., et al. (2008). Patterns of autobiographical memory loss in medial-temporal lobe amnesic patients. *Journal of Cognitive Neuroscience, 20*(8), 1490–1506. https://doi.org/10.1162/jocn.2008.20105

R Core Team. (2020). R: A language and environment for statistical computing. *R Foundation for Statistical Computing*, Vienna, Austria. https://www.R-project.org/

Tang, H., Singer, J., Ison, M. J., Pivazyan, G., Romaine, M., Frias, R., et al. (2016). Predicting episodic memory formation for movie events. *Scientific Reports, 6*(1), 1–14. https://doi.org/10.1038/srep30175

Tulving, E. (1985). Memory and consciousness. *Canadian Psychology/psychologie Canadienne, 26*(1), 1. https://doi.org/10.1037/h0080017

Tulving, E. (2002). Episodic memory: From mind to brain. *Annual Review of Psychology, 53*(1), 1–25. https://doi.org/10.1146/annurev.psych.53.100901.135114

Vogt, S., & Magnussen, S. (2007). Long-term memory for 400 pictures on a common theme. *Experimental Psychology, 54*(4), 298. https://doi.org/10.1027/1618-3169.54.4.298

Psychological Predictors of Credit Risk in Microcredit: A Microlending Case Study from Mongolia

Mandukhai Ganbat, Altantsetseg Badrakh, Byambajargal Shijir, Khosgarig Altantsatsralt, Mandakhbayar Nemekh, and Nyamdemberel Tseveendorj

Abstract Soft-data-based microcredit can bring financial inclusivity for those who are likely to be left out of financial services due to the lack of credit history or other hard data the traditional credit scoring models require. This study aims to investigate whether borrowers' credit risks are predictable through their psychological characteristics, particularly: self-control, conscientiousness, neuroticism, risk-taking, attachment, integrity, money attitude, and money management. We attempted to develop a psychometric credit scoring including the above factors (validated through Confirmatory Factor Analysis) and experimented with providing small loans for individuals using the psychometric credit scoring, through a mobile lending application, Zeely. Anyone above 18 years old who wish to borrow from Zeely and received at least 70% score on the psychometric test were eligible to become a customer. The main analyses were conducted on SPSS.25 using the linear regression and MANOVA, with the data of 12,627 borrowers who received microcredits between January 2021 and June 2022. Results revealed that money management, self-control, risk-taking, and conscientiousness predicted credit overdue days, self-control and risk-taking predicted credit default, delinquency, and normal repayment group differences, and money management, self-control, and conscientiousness predicted overall loan history-based cluster differences (or ideal and non-ideal borrowers). Male gender and younger age were related to significantly higher credit risks, yet, all four psychological factors added a significant amount of explained variances to credit overdue days after adjusting to age and gender. Therefore, it is concluded that psychological factors can be used as alternative data for credit scoring in the cultural context. Limitations, implications, and future directions are discussed.

Keywords Credit risk · Psychological factors · Microcredit · Fintech · Alternative data · Mongolia

---

M. Ganbat (✉) · A. Badrakh · B. Shijir · K. Altantsatsralt · M. Nemekh
Optimal NMAX LLC, Ulaanbaatar, Mongolia
e-mail: mandukhai@optimal.mn

N. Tseveendorj
Khatan-Suudal Invest NBFI, Ulaanbaatar, Mongolia

P. Macaulay and L. Tan (eds.), *Applied Psychology Readings*,
https://doi.org/10.1007/978-981-99-2613-8_3

1 Introduction

Financial inclusivity through soft data-based loans can bring positive changes in people's lives, especially those who are likely to be left out due to a lack of credit history and other hard data the traditional lending models require (Leong et al., 2017). The recent developments in the fintech sector—integrating technological advancements in facilitating financial services (Arner et al., 2015), such as a mobile lending application—may foster such soft-data-based loans and financial inclusivity in many countries (Menat, 2016; Muganyi et al., 2022). In Mongolia, the Financial Regulatory Commission (2021) reported that 80.4% of total borrowers, or 1.4 million people received loans through mobile lending applications in 2021, which accounted for 15.3% of the total annual loans. That is, the number of fintech borrowers in Mongolia increased 2.1 times from the previous year, or 85 out of 100 people aged 18–64 borrowed from mobile lending applications in 2021. This shows that mobile lending applications have become a popular way of requesting microcredit for Mongolians. Microcredit is defined as a very small sum of loans for individuals who are usually unable to receive such loans from commercial banking services (Hayes, 2020). However, the credit scoring systems of those fintech services in Mongolia are still inclined to use traditional demographic and financial data which are largely determined by regular full-time employment status and monthly social insurance payment amount proportionally deducted from the monthly salary. As a result, those with low or irregular income and a lack of financial history are still at risk of being discriminated against in receiving financial services. Therefore, to make fintech services more accessible, it is important to develop alternative credit scoring that is not limited to or even exclusive of those traditional data. It is also important for such an alternative scoring to accurately predict credit risk, as microcredits tend to face greater default risk than traditional loans (Serrano-Cinca et al., 2015). According to the Financial Regulatory Commission (2021), credit risks may include overdue days, credit delinquency (30–90 days overdue), and credit default (more than 90 days overdue).

Psychological factors, or the *characteristics* variable of the 5C approach of lending (Thomas, 2000), is one of the increasingly studied alternative predictors of credit risks. That is, aside from macroeconomic situations, borrower's personal characteristics, or his/her psychological, attitudinal, and behavioral characteristics tend to explain the large variances in credit risk (Ford, 2018). Previous studies argued that while financial information might predict the borrower's ability to repay, psychological information might help predict the more crucial factor, the willingness to repay (Ladas et al., 2014). There might be situations where the borrower chooses not to pay back despite their full ability to repay (Goel & Rastogi, 2021). Therefore, some bankers in England reported they put more emphasis on the applicant's personal characteristics, such as pleasantness than financial net worth when making lending decisions (Wilson et al., 2007). Also, an Indonesian fintech reported their psychological lending method produced an excellent repayment rate (Rabecca et al., 2018). However, according to Trönnberg and Hemlin (2012), neither extended access to financial information nor extensive reliance on relationship lending (i.e., soft-data-based lending method) relates to better lending decisions. Regarding the latter, they argued some borrowers might not honestly reveal their personal characteristics in high-stake situations, and loan officers' personal bias might affect rational lending decisions. Therefore, to keep objectivity and bias-free evaluation in soft-data-based lending, it is crucial to quantify personal characteristics through statistical credit scoring instead of relying on the intuitions of the loan officers. Besides, as the micro-credit demands grow larger, the loan officers cannot evaluate each loan requester's personal characteristics without an automated scoring system.

To sum up, although financial information and other market situations are predictive of loan repayment, the personal characteristics of the borrower can be used as alternative data for credit scoring, especially when there is a lack of financial history. Moreover, keeping objectivity is important when evaluating credit scores through personal characteristics.

When it comes to the relationships between personal characteristics and credit risk, the most cited, influential studies (i.e., Lea et al., 1995; Livingstone & Lunt, 1992; Tokunaga, 1993) and recent systematic reviews (i.e., Çallı & Coşkun, 2021; Goel & Rastogi, 2021) suggest various psychological, behavioral, attitudinal, and even financial literacy-related factors as the potential predictors of credit risks. In particular, Goel and Rastogi's (2021) systematic review suggested *self-control* as one of the strongest predictors of loan repayment as it inhibits and regulates impulsive spending due to emotional instability (Goel & Rastogi, 2021; Webley & Nyhus, 2001). It was repeatedly found that irresponsible, impulse-driven spending leads to over-indebtedness (Hughes, 2014; Ladas et al., 2014; Lea et al., 1995; Livingstone & Lunt, 1992). In that sense, self-control refers to self-discipline, which inhibits the impulsive behaviors (Baumeister, 2002; Shilton, 2020). Compare to other variables, self-control seems to be consistently supported by the previous studies, making it one of the soundest predictors of loan repayment.

Personality might be another potential psychological predictor of loan repayment. In particular, people who are low on *neuroticism*, but high on *conscientiousness* were found to demonstrate better repayment behaviors (Anderson et al., 2011; Chhatwani, 2022; Donnelly et al., 2012; Letkiewicz & Heckman, 2019). Neuroticism is characterized by a frequent display of negative emotions, including anxious and depressive-irritable emotions, mainly as a result of high sensitivity to environmental stimulus, while conscientiousness is characterized by a high sense of responsibility and rule obedience, making conscientious people highly reliable (Cobb-Clark & Schurer, 2012). That is, the irrational emotionality of highly neurotic people might lead to irrational, impulsive financial decisions and that may cause financial problems. As opposed to that, highly conscientious people might manage their finance better as they are more responsible. However, as the feelings of responsibility can create worries and anxiety, some people might demonstrate high neuroticism and conscientiousness simultaneously (Beckmann et al., 2010). In that instance, neuroticism can be a positive indicator of loan repayment. However, previous findings are inconsistent as some studies reported no effect of conscientiousness (Klinger et al.,

2013) and neuroticism (Ganbat et al., 2021) on loan repayment, therefore, showing the need for more studies.

Risk-taking tendency might also be responsible for credit risk. People who were high in risk-taking tended to involve in problematic behaviors such as gambling, driving under the influence, and unprotected sexual behavior (Zuckerman & Kuhlman, 2000), and such risk-taking were correlated with risky financial decisions as well (Adams & Moore, 2007). Worthy et al. (2010) found that college students who scored higher in sensation-seeking also reported a higher level of risky behaviors and more problematic financial outcomes. Similar findings were found in some non-western samples as well (Flores & Vieira, 2014). Therefore, there seems to be a relatively clear relationship between risk-taking and financial problems. However, there are still a number of studies that reported no relationship between risk-taking and indebtedness at all. For instance, Meyll and Pauls (2019) argued not the risk-taking attitude but other factors, such as the initial loan purpose, explain the over-indebtedness. Nevertheless, the majority of the previous studies supported risk-taking as a potential predictor of credit risks.

Moving further, *attachment insecurity* might also relate to the credit risk. According to Hughes (2014) and Li et al. (2020), attachment insecurity was related to emotional and irresponsible spending (similar to low self-control and high neuroticism) and lack of financial planning, thus leading to financial problems such as over-indebtedness. Adulthood attachment is conceptualized by the personal belief system about one's self and others, or the degree to which one believes in own self-worth and the trustworthiness of others (Weiss, 2006). Negative beliefs about one's self and others create a fear of rejection and loss, thus people with insecure attachment tend to have relational issues with significant others. Hughes (2014) suggested that as negative emotionality is linked with irregular and irresponsible buying, emotional distress and conflicts due to insecure attachment may result in credit risk. However, compared to the other factors, the influence of attachment on loan repayment is relatively less investigated. Moreover, some studies reported finding *integrity* to predict loan repayment (Dlugosch et al., 2018; Sohn, 2016; Wang et al., 2020). It could be that a higher level of honesty and moral principles, the elements of integrity, bring a higher willingness to repay (Goel & Rastogi, 2021). But then again, the effect of integrity was investigated less than other commonly investigated factors.

In addition to these psychological variables, financial literacy-related factors such as *money management skills* and *attitude towards money* are other potential determinants of loan repayment (see review by Çallı & Coşkun, 2021). Studies found people who carefully plan their finance, such as by using various financial management resources, and those who are confident in their financial management knowledge and skills demonstrate better repayment behaviors (Baidoo et al., 2020; Ksendzova et al., 2017; Lea et al., 1995). Moreover, Tokunaga (1993) found that problematic debtors had more problematic attitudes toward money or saw money as a source of anxiety, power, prestige, and a tool for compulsive purchasing. Such people tend to impulsively purchase and make other impulsive financial decisions to either increase the feelings of power and pleasure or to decrease the anxiety of having money, which tends to create difficulties in sticking with the loan repayment plan (Hughes, 2014).

Taken as a whole, previous studies suggested various psychological, behavioral, and attitudinal predictors of loan repayment and credit risk, although with some common limitations. First, the majority of those studies were conducted in western countries and targeted credit card users and bank loan users. Relatively little is known from the non-western samples and how these factors relate to fintech users (Baklouti, 2014). Second, the dependent variables or the chosen credit risks of the previous studies varied hugely from overdue days to credit default, and that may have produced inconsistent results. Lastly, and more importantly, very few studies developed credit scoring systems based on such psychological factors and tested them in real-life microlending practice. To the best of our knowledge, by far, there is only one fintech in Indonesia that has been successfully providing microloans based on the performance of their psychometric test (Rabecca et al., 2018). However, their model is exclusively for small and medium enterprises and entrepreneurs. Hence, there is a need to examine the effectiveness of such credit risk-predicting psychometrics in different contexts, particularly, in non-entrepreneur borrowers from a different country.

The present study intends to contribute to the literature by testing whether the proposed factors can be used as alternative data for microfinance credit scoring in the Mongolian context. To quantify these soft factors, psychometric credit scoring was developed and implemented at a local microcredit issuing mobile application Zeely,[1] by Khatan-Suudal Invest non-bank financial institution, and the relationships between the psychometric credit scores and various credit risks were examined. Based on previous studies' findings, the following hypotheses were developed.

H1: The proposed factors, self-control, conscientiousness, neuroticism, risk-taking, attachment, integrity, money attitude, and money management, will significantly predict credit overdue days.

H2: The proposed factors, self-control, conscientiousness, neuroticism, risk-taking, attachment, integrity, money attitude, and money management, will significantly differ among normal repayment, credit delinquency, and credit default groups.

H3: The proposed factors, self-control, conscientiousness, neuroticism, risk-taking, attachment, integrity, money attitude, and money management, will significantly differ among the overall loan history-based clusters (or ideal and non-ideal borrowers).

[1] Zeely is a mobile lending application that has issued around 177,400 microcredits to around 52,000 borrowers (150,000 MNT or 44 USD on average) since 2018, based on their psychometric credit scoring. There are 36 other mobile lending applications in Mongolia that lend 237,000 MNT or 70 USD on average. However, Zeely differs from other fintech by its continued attempt to develop a psychometric credit scoring system to bring inclusivity in the financial services. As of 2022, 239,000 users passed the psychometric scoring out of 355,000 attempts, and 52,000 of them proceeded to request microcredit. The share of non-performing loans in the total loan portfolio is 6.4% as of December 2022, which is 0.9% lower than the industry average.

2 Methodology

2.1 Instrument Development

To test the hypotheses, a new credit scoring instrument was developed including the proposed factors. When creating the items, the researchers (first, second, and third author) consulted previously tested western questionnaires regarding each factor and attempted to adapt the most relevant items (through face validity) in accordance with the current need. In doing so, three things were considered important. First, the items should be easily understood in the cultural context or should not be perceived as some translated sentences that have ambiguous meanings. Second, the adapted items should be worded carefully and not worded in a way that skews respondents toward a certain answer. It is especially important because based on our previous experiences (Ganbat et al., 2021), people tend to choose "the obviously right answers" when performing psychometric credit scoring and that creates a problem with data accuracy. For instance, items "*I am a highly responsible person*" or "*I manage my finance well*" often produced higher mean scores that did not relate to the loan repayment outcomes. Therefore, we aimed to prevent making similar mistakes in this study. Third, the instrument should replicate the theoretical structure of each factor. For instance, according to previous studies, three distinct components of self-control, emotional instability, emotional behavior/buying, and self-discipline seemed to predict loan repayment, while two components of money attitude, money as a source of power and prestige, and negative beliefs about money such as seeing money as a source of conflicts were related to loan repayment, and so on. As a result, the current instrument was estimated to consist of 16 subscales (Table 1). Initially, ten items were developed for each subscale, with an expectation that low quality ones will be removed resulting in fewer items. All item responses were recorded on a five-point Likert scale, ranging from 0 (not at all) to 4 (very much like me). Higher scores indicate higher self-control, conscientiousness, integrity, money management, and positive money attitude, but lower attachment insecurity, neuroticism, and risk-taking. That is, the latter three factors or the risk factors were reverse-coded to reflect a scoring scheme that higher scores indicate better performance.

Pilot study. A pilot study was conducted to examine the internal consistency and structural validity of the newly developed instrument and to get a loose orientation on the proposed factors' predictive ability of loan repayment. As of 200 Zeely borrowers who agreed to voluntarily participate and filled the survey anonymously through Survey Monkey, 170 responses were included in the data analyses after removing incomplete responses and those who failed the quality check (e.g., completed the survey too quickly or deliberately chose the same answers repeatedly). Informed consent was obtained when completing the online survey. The average age of the respondents was 25.5 (SD = 4.2), 63.7% were female and 36.3% were male.

Firstly, internal consistency reliability was analyzed using the item mean and standard deviations, item-total correlations (ITC), and Cronbach's alpha. 86 items with low ITC (<0.3) and non-normal distributions were removed. As a result, all 16

Table 1 Internal consistency reliability indices and example items

Factors		Items	ITC	Cronbach's α		Example item
Self-control	Emotional instability	7	≥0.45 and ≤0.78	0.869	0.874	"People might feel worried if they hear about things I do when in high spirits"
	Emotional buying	5	≥0.43 and ≤0.55	0.729		"Sometimes I go overboard and buy a lot without planning"
	Self-discipline	5	≥0.47 and ≤0.60	0.764		"I am having a hard time fighting with my bad habits"
Conscientiousness	Rule obedience	8	≥0.43 and ≤0.69	0.841	0.810	"I think rules and policies are meant to restrict our freedom"
	Responsibleness	5	≥0.44 and ≤0.64	0.800		"I like to take on responsible, challenging tasks"
Neuroticism	Anxiousness	3	≥0.59 and ≤0.81	0.817	0.852	"I worry about things a lot, which sometimes makes it difficult to fall asleep"
	Depressive-irritableness	5	≥0.44 and ≤0.72	0.767		"People say that when I face obstacles, I easily become irritated"

(continued)

Table 1 (continued)

Factors		Items	ITC	Cronbach's α		Example item
Risk-taking	Risk-taking	4	≥0.37 and ≤0.49	0.603	0.603	"I like trying things that excite me, even if it's a little dangerous or risky"
Attachment insecurity	Attachment insecurity	4	≥0.38 and ≤0.43	0.628	0.628	"I find it difficult to share my thoughts and feelings with my partner, although I am sure they would like it if I opened up"
Integrity	Honesty	4	≥0.34 and ≤0.35	0.630	0.667	"If I accidentally break something, I will take the blame immediately"
	Moral principles	3	≥0.39 and ≤0.50	0.649		"Sometimes I lie or cheat for better outcomes"
Money management	Unplanned spending	4	≥0.55 and ≤0.71	0.815	0.816	"Judging from the past, I spend more than I earn"
	Money management knowledge and resources	3	≥0.40 and ≤0.57	0.685		"I only save money when I need to tighten my belt"

(continued)

Table 1 (continued)

Factors		Items	ITC	Cronbach's α		Example item
	Ineffective money habits	4	≥0.40 and ≤0.55	0.688		"When I go shopping, I don't take the changes if it's just a small amount"
Money attitude	Source of power and prestige	5	≥0.48 and ≤0.74	0.816	0.668	"More money I make, the more my self-esteem will increase"
	Negative beliefs toward money	5	≥0.36 and ≤0.66	0.760		"Making more money than one's needs is not a good thing"

subscales reached a relatively acceptable level of Cronbach's alpha (ranging from 0.600 to 0.869) as shown in Table 1.

After reaching acceptable internal reliabilities, Confirmatory Factor Analyses (CFA) were performed on Amos.26 (Arbuckle, 2019) to check the factor structure and model fits. All CFA models produced a relatively acceptable fit and the anticipated number of factor structures. Particularly, attachment insecurity, risk-taking, and integrity produced the most acceptable fit indices, however, self-control, conscientiousness, neuroticism, money management, and money attitude produced less acceptable fit indices but many of the requirements of an acceptable model were demonstrated in each model (Table 2). All items were loading above 0.40 as recommended by Stevens (1992), except for an item of negative attitudes toward money and an item of risk-taking. Removal of those two items did not produce significantly improved model fits, thus, the items were retained. Therefore, the final version of the instrument consisted of 74 items as shown in Table 1. Moreover, all latent variables were significantly correlated ($p < 0.01$), at low to moderate levels (from 0.353 to 0.633), except for money attitude and conscientiousness scales where no significant correlations were found among their subscales.

Lastly, the pilot study's participants were asked "*Have you ever failed to pay your loan on time?*" to roughly examine the proposed factors' predictive abilities on loan repayment (i.e., due to anonymity, their data recorded on the Zeely database were not usable). 29.4% answered "yes", and 70.6% answered "no". For participants who answered "yes", 92% repaid in less than 30 days overdue or before the loan history proceeded to delinquency, and 8% paid in more than 30 days. As shown in

Table 2 Fit indices of CFA models

Model	Factor structure	I2	DF	Sig	CFI	TLI	RMSEA
Self-control	3	160.349	113	$p < 0.002$	0.910	0.892	0.071
Conscientiousness	2	85.541	64	$p < 0.037$	0.938	0.924	0.063
Neuroticism	2	31.788	19	$p < 0.033$	0.948	0.924	0.080
Risk-taking	1	0.729	2	$p < 0.695$	1.000	1.114	0.000
Attachment	1	1.015	2	$p < 0.602$	1.000	1.094	0.000
Integrity	2	4.674	13	$p < 0.982$	1.000	1.226	0.000
Money management	3	45.098	41	$p < 0.001$	0.983	0.977	0.034
Money attitude	2	49.480	34	$p < 0.042$	0.937	0.916	0.074

Note I2 = Chi square, DF = degree of freedom, CFI = comparative fit index, TLI = Tucker-Lewis Index, RMSEA = root mean square error of approximation

Table 3, significant differences were found between participants who always pay their loans on time and those who occasionally pay late regarding all factors, except for emotional instability, risk-taking, moral principles, and seeing money as power and prestige. That is, the pilot study's participants tended to evaluate themselves as relatively emotionally stable, have higher moral principles, and relatively higher in risk-taking and seeing money as a source of power and prestige, regardless of their loan repayment behavior. Higher risk-taking could be due to the relatively young mean age (25.5) and seeing money as a source of power and prestige could be a cultural effect that relatively lower economic growth and higher corruption rate (Sergelenbat, 2021) of Mongolia might be producing this effect. Moreover, some of these significant differences in t-tests became insignificant in the multivariate analysis. The emotional instability (p = 0.041, odds ratio = 2.94, SE = 0.527), emotional buying (p = 0.002, odds ratio = 0.155, SE = 0.613), self-discipline (p = 0.021, odds ratio = 0.285, SE = 0.544), moral principles (p = 0.012, odds ratio = 3.06, SE = 0.444), responsibleness (p = 0.014, odds ratio = 3.71, SE = 0.536), and unplanned spending (p = 0.000, odds ratio = 0.128, SE = 0.510) remained significant, suggesting these might be the strongest predictors in loan repayment in the cultural context. Nevertheless, no scale or subscale was removed based on the pilot results.

2.2 Participants and Procedure

Around 15,000 people received microcredits through the Zeely mobile lending application between January 2021 and June 2022 based on their performance on the above instrument. New borrowers or those who used the loan for less than 28 days were excluded from analyses due to lack of loan repayment data. As a result, data of 12,627 borrowers were analyzed. The consent was taken from each borrower when signing the loan agreement that their data could be used anonymously for research purposes.

Table 3 T-test statistics of pilot study

		Mean (SD) Group 1	Mean (SD) Group 2	t	Hedges' *g*
Self-control	Emotional instability (R)	2.71(0.73)	2.53(0.71)	1.47	0.25
	Emotional buying (R)	2.59(0.58)	2.20(0.55)	4.05***	0.68
	Self-discipline	2.25(0.70)	1.88(0.68)	3.15**	0.53
Conscientiousness	Rule obedience	2.64(0.60)	2.29(0.69)	3.38***	0.55
	Responsibleness	2.39(0.61)	2.18(0.68)	2.00*	0.33
Neuroticism	Anxiousness (R)	1.91(0.87)	1.58(0.78)	2.32*	0.39
	Depressive-irritableness (R)	1.89(0.58)	1.60(0.62)	2.84**	0.49
Risk-taking	Risk-taking (R)	2.05(0.59)	2.04(0.68)	0.13	0.01
Attachment insecurity	Attachment insecurity (R)	2.73(0.58)	2.38(0.73)	3.33**	0.56
Integrity	Honesty	2.70(0.56)	2.43(0.55)	2.96**	0.48
	Moral principles	2.60(0.83)	2.54(0.86)	0.37	0.07
Money management	Unplanned spending (R)	2.62(0.67)	1.92(0.66)	6.24***	1.04
	Money management knowledge and resources	2.25(0.76)	1.90(0.90)	2.50*	0.43
	Ineffective money habits (R)	2.74(0.54)	2.36(0.86)	3.52**	0.58
Money attitude	Source of power and prestige (R)	2.08(0.77)	1.90(0.73)	1.40	0.21
	Negative beliefs toward money (R)	2.75(0.64)	2.52(0.51)	2.19*	0.38

Note Group 1 = never failed to pay on time, Group 2 = occasional failure to pay on time, SD = standard deviation, df = degree of freedom, $0.00 < g > 0.20$ = no effect, $0.20 < g > 0.50$ = small effect, $0.50 < g > 0.80$ = medium effect, $g \geq 0.80$ = large effect, R = reversed (for example, higher scores in emotional instability represent lower original score), * $p < 0.05$, ** $p < 0.01$, *** $p < 0.001$, degree of freedom for t test = 168

The average age of the borrowers included in the data analyses was 30 (SD = 7.1, ranging from 19 to 79). 58.2% were female, and 41.8% were male.

In evaluating the credit scoring, users were asked to respond to one randomly selected item from each subscale or a total of 16 items, as the total instrument was considered too long. Resultantly, the credit scoring was able to be calculated within less than three minutes. All items were coded in a way that lower scores indicate a higher likelihood of credit risks. In other words, if the user selected "4" or "very much like me" on negative items such as "*People say that when I face obstacles, I easily become irritated*", the score was reversed to "0". Users who received at least 70% of the total score were considered as passed the scoring and therefore received the microcredits (i.e., as microcredits face greater default rate, applying cut-off score was necessary). That is, the credit score was calculated by the sum of the scores of all 16 subscales. As a quality check, the users were asked to enable their front camera while responding to the items. Lastly, users' demographic information, age and gender, was asked, only for research purposes.

2.3 Data Analysis

Data analyses were performed on SPSS. 25 (IBM Corp, 2017). To test H1, or whether the proposed factors predict credit overdue days, linear regression analyses were carried out for each proposed factor, adjusting for age and gender. When there is more than one loan account per borrower (meaning the borrower received more than one loan), the maximum overdue day was used, and the overdue days ranged from 0 to 464 (Mean = 26.38, SD = 62.15, median = 2.00).

For H2 and H3, MANOVA tests were carried out to analyze the differences between the groups regarding the independent variables. For H2, three groups were created using maximum overdue days, normal repayment group (i.e., zero to 29 days overdue), credit delinquency group (i.e., 30 to 90 days overdue), and credit default group (i.e., more than 90 days overdue). 10,316 borrowers or 81.7% were classified into the normal repayment group (61.0% were females and 39.0% were males), 1106 borrowers, or 8.8% were classified into the credit delinquency group (44.6% were females and 55.4% were males), and 1205 borrowers or 9.5% were classified into credit default group (45.9% were females and 54.1% were males).

For H3, four groups were created based on their overall history of loan repayment. That is, while H2 groups were created based on each borrower's "worst" possible repayment history, H3 attempted to cluster the borrowers based on their overall loan history on Zeely. Particularly, (1) total loan accounts, (2) total overdue accounts, (3) total overdue days, and (4) total number of days that the borrower has used the loan were used to build the cluster model on R version 4.2.1 (R Core Team, 2013). Before comparing the different variables, the numeric variables were standardized. The k-means method was applied in building clusters, and to determine the number of optimal clusters, the elbow method was used. Elbow is a simple visual technique in which the number of clusters is determined by the "elbow" shaped point (Humaira & Rasyidah, 2020). As shown in Fig. 1, larger value differences were observed between Cluster 1, 2, 3, and 4, and starting from Cluster 4 to 5 small differences were observed, making the elbow point. Hence, the visualization demonstrated that the optimal number of clusters was four.

As shown in Table 4, 838 borrowers (6.6%) were classified into Cluster 1, the non-ideal borrowers, with the highest total overdue days (M = 231.78) and the lowest total account (M = 3.24). 2318 borrowers (18.4%) were classified into Cluster 2, or the regular borrowers, with a higher number of total accounts (M = 8.17) and relatively lower total overdue days (M = 31.40). 6664 borrowers (52.8%) were classified into Cluster 3, the new borrowers with thinner history, with even lower total overdue days (M = 12.56) and relatively lower total accounts (M = 4.77). Lastly, 2807 borrowers (22.2%) were classified into Cluster 4, the ideal borrowers, with the lowest total

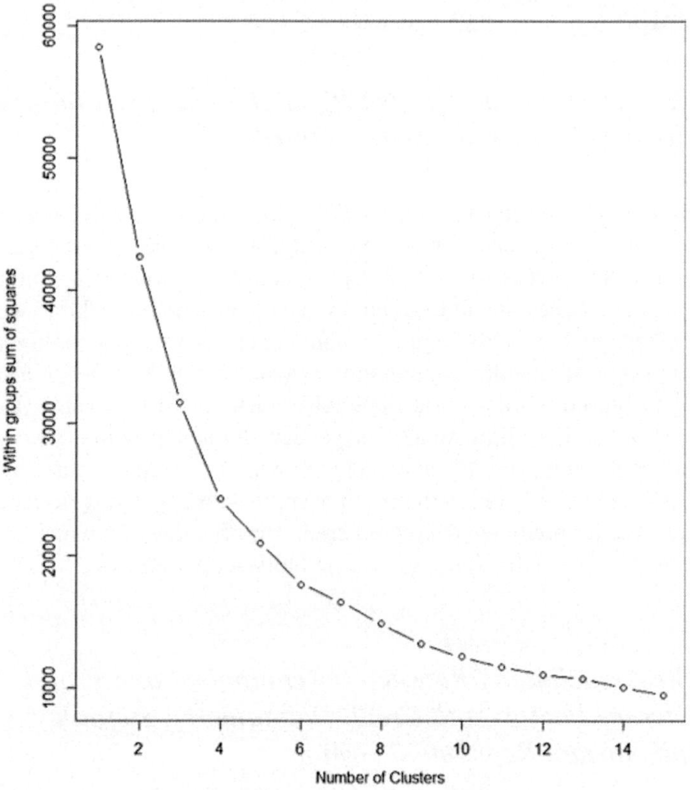

Fig. 1 Elbow method determining the optimal number of clusters

overdue days (M = 3.68) and the highest total accounts (M = 15.55). In other words, Cluster 4 borrowers use the loan application most frequently and almost always repay before the due date.

Table 4 Clusters' descriptive

Cluster	Given names	Total overdue accounts (M)	Total overdue days (M)	Total accounts (M)	Total use days (M)	N	%
1	Non-ideal borrowers	1.71	231.78	3.24	340.78	838	6.6%
2	Regular borrowers	3.51	31.40	8.17	324.45	2318	18.4%
3	New borrowers	0.80	12.56	4.77	151.33	6664	52.8%
4	Ideal borrowers	0.63	3.68	15.55	379.35	2807	22.2%

3 Results

3.1 The Associations Between Psychological and Financial Literacy Factors and Credit Overdue days

Adjusting for age and gender, emotional buying, rule obedience, responsibleness, risk-taking, and money management knowledge and resources were negatively associated with credit overdue days, as shown in Table 5. Negative associations were due to all negative variables (in this case, emotional buying and risk-taking) were reverse-coded. That is, lower levels of emotional buying and risk-taking but higher levels of rule obedience, responsibleness, and money management knowledge and resources predicted decreased credit overdue days. All associations added a significant amount of effect size after controlling for age and gender, although the effect sizes were small. Other variables had no significant association with the credit overdue days. Age and gender both significantly predicted credit overdue days negatively that increased age and female gender predicted decreased credit overdue days. In which, the effect of gender was stronger. Therefore, H1 was partially supported.

3.2 The Associations Between Psychological and Financial Literacy Factors and Credit Delinquency, Default, and Normal Repayment Groups

The multivariate analysis supported there was a significant effect of the psychological and financial literacy-related independent variables on the group differences (Wilks' Lambda = 0.996, F (32, 25,218) = 1.44, $p = 0.049$, partial $\eta^2 = 0.002$). As shown in Table 5, the group differences occurred regarding emotional buying and risk-taking, although both with small effect sizes (partial $\eta^2 = 0.004$). The effect sizes estimate the magnitude of the differences between groups. In this case, the partial eta squared statistics are telling us there were very small effects (<0.06) of the independent variables, emotional buying and risk-taking, on the dependent variable or the group differences. Therefore, emotional buying, Tukey–Kramer's post hoc test showed a significant difference was observed between the normal repayment group and credit default group (mean difference = 0.031, $p = 0.016$) that the normal repayment group was lower on emotional buying than the credit default group, although the difference was small. The credit delinquency group did not significantly differ from both credit default and normal repayment groups. For risk-taking, differences were observed between the normal repayment and credit default groups (mean difference = 0.023, $p = 0.042$) as well as between credit delinquency and credit default groups (mean difference = 0.034, $p = 0.024$). That is, the normal repayment group was lower than the credit delinquency group, while the credit delinquency group was lower than the credit default group on risk-taking. No mean difference was observed between

Table 5 Associations between psychological and financial literacy predictors and credit risks

		M (SD)	Credit overdue days		Credit delinquency, default, and normal repayment group differences		Overall loan history-based cluster differences	
			β	R^2 and F changes[A]	F	Partial η^2	F	Partial η^2
Demographic factors								
Age (continuous)		30.82(7.1)	*−0.030****		*17.77****	0.003	*16.90****	0.004
Gender (male = 0, female = 1)		0.58(0.49)	*−0.099****		*97.95***	0.015	*59.77****	0.014
Psychological factors								
Self-control	Emotional instability (R)	2.84(0.91)	−0.007		2.53		0.57	
	Emotional buying (R)	2.68(0.93)	*−0.068***	0.005(9.33)**	*4.04***	0.004	*5.26****	0.009
	Self-discipline	2.49(1.01)	−0.015		0.814		0.70	
Conscientiousness	Rule obedience	2.59(1.03)	*−0.071***	0.005(9.38)**	2.51		*2.82**	0.006
	Responsibleness	2.79(0.83)	*−0.059**	0.004(2.45)*	1.33		0.97	
Neuroticism	Anxiousness (R)	2.05(1.04)	0.002		0.57		1.78	
	Depressive-irritableness (R)	2.55(0.97)	0.001		1.44		0.10	
Risk-taking	Risk-taking (R)	1.87(0.98)	*−0.056**	0.003(3.96)*	*3.89**	0.004	1.60	
Attachment insecurity	Attachment insecurity (R)	3.14(1.14)	−0.033		0.24		1.13	
Integrity	Honesty	2.75(1.00)	−0.031		0.76		0.03	
	Moral principles	3.11(1.09)	−0.023		1.31		1.52	
Financial literacy factors								
Money management	Unplanned spending (R)	2.47(0.85)	−0.021		0.56		0.65	

(continued)

Table 5 (continued)

		M (SD)	Credit overdue days		Credit delinquency, default, and normal repayment group differences		Overall loan history-based cluster differences	
			β	R^2 and *F* changes[A]	*F*	Partial η^2	*F*	Partial η^2
	Money management knowledge and resources	2.30(0.95)	*−0.069***	0.005(8.86)**	0.97		*2.76**	0.008
	Ineffective money habits (R)	2.74(1.10)	−0.036		0.56		1.05	
Money attitude	Source of power and prestige (R)	1.96(0.99)	−0.032		1.32		0.42	
	Negative beliefs toward money (R)	2.36(1.07)	−0.038		0.74		0.61	

R = reversed, A = adjusting for sex and gender, M = mean, SD = standard deviation, * $p < 0.05$. **$p < 0.01$. ***$p < 0.001$, degree of freedom for F test = 2, 12,624 the normal repayment and credit delinquency groups regarding risk-taking. Both age and gender differences were observed. Regarding age, the normal repayment group significantly differed from both credit delinquency (mean difference = 0.95, p = 0.000) and credit default groups (mean difference = 1.00, p = 0.000). That is, the mean age of the normal repayment group was older than both credit delinquency and default groups. No age difference was observed between credit delinquency and default groups. Significantly more females were in the normal repayment group than credit delinquency (mean difference = 0.16, p = 0.000) and credit default groups (mean difference = 0.15, p = 0.000). No difference was observed between credit delinquency and default groups in terms of gender. The effect size of the gender (partial $\eta^2 = 0.015$) was slightly higher than age (partial $\eta^2 = 0.003$). Therefore, H2 was partially supported.

3.3 The Associations Between Psychological and Financial Literacy Factors and Overall Loan History-Based Clusters

The multivariate analysis supported that there was a significant effect of the psychological and financial literacy-related independent variables on the cluster differences (Wilks' Lambda = 0.995, F (48, 37,500) = 1.32, p = 0.050, partial η^2 = 0.002). As shown in Table 5, significant differences were observed among clusters regarding emotional buying, rule obedience, and money management knowledge and resources, although with small effect sizes (partial η^2 ranged from 0.006 to 0.009). In other words, these variables had only small effects in terms of determining the differences between these groups. Tukey–Kramer's test showed that, for emotional buying, significant differences were observed between cluster 1 (non-ideal borrowers) and cluster 3 (new borrowers), that cluster 1 borrowers were higher on emotional buying than cluster 3 borrowers (mean difference = −0.04, p = 0.012), and between cluster 2 (regular borrowers with occasional overdue repayments) and cluster 3 (new borrowers) that cluster 2 borrowers were higher on emotional buying than cluster 3 borrowers (mean difference = −0.03, p = 0.013). No other differences were observed regarding emotional buying. Regarding rule obedience, the significant difference observed between cluster 1 (non-ideal borrowers) and cluster 3 (new borrowers) that new borrowers were slightly higher on rule obedience (mean difference = −0.02, p = 0.050). Regarding money management knowledge and resources, the significant difference observed between cluster 1 (non-ideal borrowers) and cluster 3 (new borrowers) that new borrowers were slightly higher on money management knowledge and resources (mean difference = −0.02, p = 0.05). Both age and gender significantly differed among clusters. Particularly, the mean age of cluster 1 (non-ideal) borrowers was significantly younger than cluster 3 (new borrowers, mean difference = −0.72, p = 0.030) and cluster 4 (ideal borrowers, mean difference =

-1.25, $p = 0.000$). Cluster 2 (regular borrowers with occasional overdue repayments) had significantly younger mean age than cluster 3 (new borrowers, mean difference $= -0.77$, $p = 0.000$) and cluster 4 (ideal borrowers, mean difference $= -1.31$, $p = 0.000$). Cluster 3 (new borrowers) had significantly younger mean age than cluster 4 (ideal borrowers, mean difference $= -0.54$, $p = 0.000$), or cluster 4 (ideal borrowers) had significantly older mean age than all other clusters. Cluster 1 (non-ideal borrowers) had significantly more males than cluster 2 (regular borrowers, mean difference $= -0.11$, $p = 0.000$), cluster 3 (new borrowers, mean difference $= -0.10$, $p = 0.000$), and cluster 4 (ideal borrowers, mean difference $= -0.22$, $p = 0.000$). Cluster 2 (regular borrowers) and 3 (new borrowers) had significantly more males than cluster 4 (ideal borrowers, mean difference $= -0.11$ and -0.12, $p = 0.000$). Therefore, H3 was partially supported.

4 Discussion

This study investigated the predictive abilities of psychological (and some financial literacy) variables in credit risks in the Mongolian context. Particularly, this study was interested in whether psychometric credit scoring, including self-control, conscientiousness, neuroticism, risk-taking, attachment, integrity, money management, and money attitude would predict microcredit risks, therefore be successfully used as an alternative scoring in the microlending practice. As of 12,627 borrowers who received microcredits between January 2021 and June 2022, 10,316 borrowers, or 81.6%, repaid the loan within the due day or before reaching credit delinquency, 1106 borrowers, or 8.8%, repaid in 30 to 90 days overdue, and remaining 1205 borrowers, or 9.5%, reached credit default or did not pay back within 90 days overdue. The fact that every eight out of 10 borrowers paid back, mostly on time, shows that the psychometric credit scoring was largely successful.

Particularly, the analyses showed that the emotional buying subscale of self-control, rule obedience and responsibleness subscales of conscientiousness, risk-taking, money management knowledge, and resources subscale of money management had significant effects on loan repayment. Among these, emotional buying was the only factor that predicted each risk respectively, or higher scores on emotional buying were related to increased overdue days, and increased risk for credit default, therefore, more likely to fall for cluster 1 or non-ideal borrowers' group. This finding replicates previous findings, in another country, that people who lack self-control tend to be more impulsive and make emotional financial decisions such as emotional buying which results in loan repayment difficulties (Baumeister, 2002; Goel & Rastogi, 2021). However, it is possible that why some people are more prone to emotional buying than others can be explained through other factors, such as social comparison than self-control (Lea et al., 1995). It was suggested in previous studies that some people may adopt an inappropriate reference group and compare themselves with people who have more economic resources than them, which puts them in danger of overspending (Lunt & Livingstone, 1991). In other words, it might be that the feelings of comparing one's self with more fortunate others may cause impulsivity to buy things one cannot afford. Yet, even in that case, self-control seems still to play an important role to regulate such impulsive desire to "keep up with the Joneses". Moreover, the finding also appears to support Ottaviani and Vandone (2011), who suggested emotional buying and over-indebtedness more relate to unsecured loans such as credit card use and personal loans. That is, for the borrowers of this study especially for the regular borrowers, the microcredits might be serving as consumer credit, hence, might explain why emotional buying was found to predict various credit risks while most of the other factors failed to do so. In the future, it might need to be investigated how the purpose and usage of such microcredits moderate or mediate the associations found in this study.

Furthermore, in line with Anderson et al. (2011) and Ganbat et al. (2021), current findings suggest conscientious personality indeed predicts better loan repayment or obeying rules and being responsible are likely to be important characteristics that need to be assessed when deciding whether to grant credit. Moreover, higher risk-taking was associated with increased credit overdue days and increased chances of credit delinquency and default, in line with previous findings from other countries (Adams & Moore, 2007; Flores & Vieira, 2014; Worthy et al., 2010). The association between risk-taking and credit risks was largely explained by Zuckerman's (1979) sensation-seeking theory. Zuckerman argues that although sensation-seeking is a normal, genetically influenced personality trait that is characterized by the need for varied, novel, and complex experiences and willingness to take social and physical risks for the sake of such sensations, the maladaptive form of sensation-seeking may cause problematic risky behaviors such as extreme gambling, substance abuse, unsafe sexual activities, and so on. Such behaviors were related to problematic financial outcomes as well (Adams & Moore, 2007). That is, people with higher risk-taking tendencies may excessively abuse their credit for the sake of high arousal experiences, and that perhaps cause problems with loan repayment.

Lastly, increased money management knowledge and resources predicted decreased credit overdue days and decreased chances of clustering into non-ideal borrowers. According to Letkiewicz and Fox (2014), as financial products are becoming more and more complex, most people find basic financial concepts hard to understand, which may diminish one's chances of financially thriving. To put it simply, people may overuse or mismanage their credits because of a lack of financial literacy. On the other hand, increased knowledge providing on how to manage one's money effectively perhaps through the use of various financial management tools may increase one's ability and confidence in money management and eventually have a positive effect on loan repayment (Baidoo et al., 2020; Ksendzova et al., 2017; Lea et al., 1995).

However, the effects of those four factors on credit risks were rather small, and neuroticism, attachment insecurity, integrity, and money attitude did not associate with credit risks at all. Therefore, other factors not included in this study may explain credit risks more effectively. Particularly, younger age and male gender predicted all credit risks much more strongly than the psychological factors. Suggesting that these demographic variables may need to be considered as important factors in soft-data-based lending. However, there are other perhaps more reasonable explanations as to why the proposed factors did not have large effects on the loan repayment outcomes. First, there is a possibility that borrowers rated themselves as positively as they could in the psychometric credit scoring, therefore, producing rather small differences between individuals. If a similar questionnaire was taken in low-stake situations or unrelatedly to the lending decisions, much higher variances may have been found. Second, the fact that all borrowers included in the analyses received 70% or above scores in the psychometric credit scoring may also account for the small individual differences. In case people who received lower credit scores were granted microcredits and were included in the analyses, the results might have been different. Nevertheless, the 81.6% success rate found in this study suggests psychological variables can be used as reliable alternative data in predicting credit risk in microcredit settings, especially when used in combination with demographic data.

5 Limitations, Implications, and Future Directions

The main limitation of the current study is it did not take potential confounding effects that could affect loan repayment into account. Particularly, the inflation rate increased significantly in Mongolia in recent years (according to Asian Development Bank 2022, the inflation rate was 7.10% in 2021 that was 3.41% increase from 2020, and forecasted at 14.7% in 2022 that is a 7.6% increase from 2021). As the macroeconomic situation is one of the most important factors that determine the loan repayment rate (Ford, 2018), the increased inflation rate may have caused some difficulties for some people to pay back their debt. Moreover, sudden adverse life events, such as illness and the death of significant someone, are other potential confounding effects that may have influenced the loan repayment rate (Tokunaga, 1993). These effects are encouraged to be controlled in further studies. The second limitation is that as this study did not grant loan for those who failed the psychometric credit scoring, the loan repayment rate differences between those who failed and passed the credit scoring is not computable. Resultantly, it is unknown whether the loan repayment rate of 81.6% was purely due to the performance on the psychometric credit scoring. Other factors might have influenced the loan repayment rate. For instance, it is possible that the low amount of microcredit (44 USD on average) was rather easier to repay than a more significant amount of loans. Lastly, the variables included in this study did not offer a comprehensive explanatory model, or the relationships and interactions between the predictors were not investigated.

Despite these limitations, this study is one of the first that experimented with using psychometric data for credit scoring. Previous studies showed enough that psychological factors relate to credit risks, however, very few developed psychological data-based statistical credit scoring and used it in real-life lending practice (Rabecca et al., 2018). Attempts to quantify borrowers' soft information have become crucial, especially when the lending market is shifting from traditional credit scoring systems to alternative data-based more inclusive credit scorings.

Future studies are encouraged to investigate the relationships among the predictors and perhaps how they interact with demographic backgrounds, for developing an explanatory model of psychological determinants of credit risk. Future studies are also encouraged to control the confounding effects of macroeconomic situations and adverse life events, and examine whether the proposed psychological factors add significant predictive ability beyond those effects.

6 Conclusion

This study investigated the predictive abilities of some psychological and financial literacy-related factors in credit risks using data from 12,627 microcredit borrowers. The results showed that 81.6% of total borrowers who received microcredits through the psychometric credit scoring paid back their debt mostly on time or within a few days of the due day. Credit risks were negatively predicted by rule obedience, responsibleness, and money management knowledge and resources, and positively predicted by emotional buying and risk-taking. Age and gender both predicted credit risks. Hence, it is concluded that psychological variables can be used as alternative data for credit scoring in the microfinancing sector in Mongolia. The combination of psychological, financial literacy-related, and demographic factors might result in a more accurate prediction of credit risk.

References

Adams, T., & Moore, M. (2007). High-risk he alth and credit behavior among 18-to 25-year-old college students. *Journal of American College Health, 56*(2), 101–108. https://doi.org/10.3200/JACH.56.2.101-108

Anderson, J., Burks, S., DeYoung, C., & Rustichini, A. (2011). Toward the integration of personality theory and decision theory in the explanation of economic behavior. In *Unpublished manuscript. Presented at the IZA workshop: Cognitive and non-cognitive skills.* https://doi.org/10.1016/j.socec.2016.04.019

Anuradha, N. (2020). Factors affecting non-performing loan portfolio in micro-lending: Evidence from Sri Lanka. *International Journal of Science and Research (IJSR), ResearchGate Impact Factor (2018): 0.28| SJIF (2018), 7*

Arbuckle, J. L. (2019). Amos (Version 26.0) [Computer Program]. Chicago: IBM SPSS.

Arner, D. W., Barberis, J., & Buckley, R. P. (2015). The evolution of fintech: A new post-crisis paradigm. *Georgetown Journal of International Law, 47*, 1271.

Asian Development Bank. (September 2022). Asian Development Outlook 2022 Update. https://www.adb.org/countries/mongolia/economy

Baidoo, S. T., Yusif, H., & Ayesu, E. K. (2020). Improving loan repayment in Ghana: Does financial literacy matter? *Cogent Economics & Finance, 8*(1), 1787693. https://doi.org/10.1080/23322039.2020.1787693

Baklouti, I. (2014). A psychological approach to microfinance credit scoring via a classification and regression tree. *Intelligent Systems in Accounting, Finance and Management, 21*(4), 193–208. https://doi.org/10.1002/isaf.1355

Baumeister, R. F. (2002). Yielding to temptation: Self-control failure, impulsive purchasing, and consumer behavior. *Journal of Consumer Research, 28*(4), 670–676. https://doi.org/10.1086/338209

Beckmann, N., Wood, R. E., & Minbashian, A. (2010). It depends how you look at it: On the relationship between neuroticism and conscientiousness at the within-and the between-person levels of analysis. *Journal of Research in Personality, 44*(5), 593–601. https://doi.org/10.1016/j.jrp.2010.07.004

Çallı, B. A., & Coşkun, E. (2021). A longitudinal systematic review of credit risk assessment and credit default predictors. *SAGE Open, 11*(4), 21582440211061332. https://doi.org/10.1177/21582440211061332

Chhatwani, M. (2022). Mortgage delinquency during COVID-19: Do financial literacy and personality traits matter? *International Journal of Bank Marketing*. https://doi.org/10.1108/IJBM-05-2021-0215

Cobb-Clark, D. A., & Schurer, S. (2012). The stability of big-five personality traits. *Economics Letters, 115*(1), 11–15. https://doi.org/10.1016/j.econlet.2011.11.015

Dlugosch, T. J., Klinger, B., Frese, M., & Klehe, U. C. (2018). Personality-based selection of entrepreneurial borrowers to reduce credit risk: Two studies on prediction models in low-and high-stakes settings in developing countries. *Journal of Organizational Behavior, 39*(5), 612–628. https://doi.org/10.1002/job.2236

Donnelly, G., Iyer, R., & Howell, R. T. (2012). The big five personality traits, material values, and financial well-being of self-described money managers. *Journal of Economic Psychology, 33*(6), 1129–1142. https://doi.org/10.1016/j.joep.2012.08.001

Financial Regulatory Commission. (2021). Financial industry overview. http://www.frc.mn/resource/frc/Document/2022/05/19/y1j3ndbaqwnzmitq/Toim%202022%20I%20final.pdf

Flores, S. A. M., & Vieira, K. M. (2014). Propensity toward indebtedness: An analysis using behavioral factors. *Journal of Behavioral and Experimental Finance, 3*, 1–10. https://doi.org/10.1016/j.jbef.2014.05.001

Ford, J. (2018). *The indebted society: Credit and default in the 1980s*. Routledge.

Ganbat, M., Batbaatar, E., Bazarragchaa, G., Ider, T., Gantumur, E., Dashkhorol, L., & Namsrai, O. E. (2021). Effect of psychological factors on credit risk: A case study of the microlending service in Mongolia. *Behavioral Sciences, 11*(4), 47. https://doi.org/10.3390/bs11040047

Goel, A., & Rastogi, S. (2021). Understanding the impact of borrowers' behavioural and psychological traits on credit default: Review and conceptual model. *Review of Behavioral Finance*. https://doi.org/10.1108/RBF-03-2021-0051

Hayes, A. (2020, November 30). *Microcredits: Definition, how it works, loan terms*. Investopedia. https://www.investopedia.com/terms/m/microcredit.asp

Hughes, D. J. (2014). *Accounting for individual differences in financial behaviour: The role of personality in insurance claims and credit behaviour*. The University of Manchester (United Kingdom).

Humaira, H., & Rasyidah, R. (2020). Determining the appropiate cluster number using Elbow method for K-Means algorithm. In *Proceedings of the 2nd Workshop on Multidisciplinary and Applications (WMA)*

IBM Corp. (2017). IBM SPSS statistics for windows, version 25.0. Armonk, NY: IBM Corp.

Klinger, B., Khwaja, A. I., & Del Carpio, C. (2013). *Enterprising psychometrics and poverty reduction* (Vol. 860). Springer.

Ksendzova, M., Donnelly, G. E., & Howell, R. T. (2017). A brief money management scale and its associations with personality, financial health, and hypothetical debt repayment. *Journal of Financial Counseling and Planning, 28*(1), 62–75. https://doi.org/10.1891/1052-3073.28.1.62

Ladas, A., Aickelin, U., Ferguson, E., & Garibaldi, J. (2014, December). A data mining framework to model consumer indebtedness with psychological factors. In *2014 IEEE International*

Conference on Data Mining Workshop (pp. 150–157). IEEE. https://doi.org/10.1109/ICDMW.2014.148

Lea, S. E., Webley, P., & Walker, C. M. (1995). Psychological factors in consumer debt: Money management, economic socialization, and credit use. *Journal of Economic Psychology, 16*(4), 681–701. https://doi.org/10.1016/0167-4870(95)00013-4

Leong, C., Tan, B., Xiao, X., Tan, F. T. C., & Sun, Y. (2017). Nurturing a FinTech ecosystem: The case of a youth microloan startup in China. *International Journal of Information Management, 37*(2), 92–97. https://doi.org/10.1016/j.ijinfomgt.2016.11.006

Letkiewicz, J. C., & Fox, J. J. (2014). Conscientiousness, financial literacy, and asset accumulation of young adults. *Journal of Consumer Affairs, 48*(2), 274–300. https://doi.org/10.1111/joca.12040

Letkiewicz, J. C., & Heckman, S. J. (2019). Repeated payment delinquency among young adults in the United States. *International Journal of Consumer Studies, 43*(5), 417–428. https://doi.org/10.1111/ijcs.12522

Li, X., Curran, M. A., LeBaron, A. B., Serido, J., & Shim, S. (2020). Romantic attachment orientations, financial behaviors, and life outcomes among young adults: A mediating analysis of a college cohort. *Journal of Family and Economic Issues, 41*(4), 658–671. https://doi.org/10.1007/s10834-020-09664-1

Livingstone, S. M., & Lunt, P. K. (1992). Predicting personal debt and debt repayment: Psychological, social and economic determinants. *Journal of Economic Psychology, 13*(1), 111–134. https://doi.org/10.1016/0167-4870(92)90055-C

Lunt, P. K., & Livingstone, S. M. (1991). Everyday explanations for personal debt: A network approach. *British Journal of Social Psychology, 30*(4), 309–323. https://doi.org/10.1111/j.2044-8309.1991.tb00948.x

Menat, R. (2016). Why we're so excited about FinTech. In *The fintech book: The financial technology handbook for investors, entrepreneurs and visionaries* (pp. 10–12). https://doi.org/10.1002/9781119218906.ch2

Meyll, T., & Pauls, T. (2019). The gender gap in over-indebtedness. *Finance Research Letters, 31*. https://doi.org/10.1016/j.frl.2018.12.007

Muganyi, T., Yan, L., Yin, Y., Sun, H., Gong, X., & Taghizadeh-Hesary, F. (2022). Fintech, regtech, and financial development: Evidence from China. *Financial Innovation, 8*(1), 1–20. https://doi.org/10.1186/s40854-021-00313-6

Ottaviani, C., & Vandone, D. (2011). Impulsivity and household indebtedness: Evidence from real life. *Journal of Economic Psychology, 32*(5), 754–761. https://doi.org/10.1016/j.joep.2011.05.002

R Core Team (2013). R: A language and environment for statistical computing. R Foundation for Statistical Computing, Vienna, Austria. http://www.R-project.org/

Rabecca, H., Atmaja, N. D., & Safitri, S. (2018). Psychometric credit scoring in indonesia microfinance industry: A case study in pt amartha mikro fintek. In *The 3rd International Conference on Management in Emerging Markets (ICMEM 2018)* (pp. 620–631)

Sergelenbat, A. (2021). *An effort to establish effective corporate governance practice, impacts on corruption, and sustainable development in developing countries: A case of Mongolia* (Doctoral dissertation, University of the West of Scotland).

Serrano-Cinca, C., Gutiérrez-Nieto, B., & López-Palacios, L. (2015). Determinants of default in P2P lending. *PloS One, 10*(10), e0139427. https://doi.org/10.1371/journal.pone.0139427

Shilton, D., Breski, M., Dor, D., & Jablonka, E. (2020). Human social evolution: Self-domestication or self control? *Frontiers in Psychology, 11*, 134. https://doi.org/10.3389/fpsyg.2020.00134

Sohn, S. Y. (2016). Fuzzy analytic hierarchy process applied to technology credit scorecard considering entrepreneurs' psychological and behavioral attributes. *Journal of Intelligent & Fuzzy Systems, 30*(4), 2349–2364. https://doi.org/10.3233/IFS-152005

Stevens, J. (1992). *Applied multivariate statistics for the social sciences* (2nd ed.). Erlbaum.

Thomas, L. C. (2000). A survey of credit and behavioural scoring: Forecasting financial risk of lending to consumers. *International Journal of Forecasting, 16*(2), 149–172. https://doi.org/10.1016/S0169-2070(00)00034-0

Tokunaga, H. (1993). The use and abuse of consumer credit: Application of psychological theory and research. *Journal of Economic Psychology, 14*(2), 285–316. https://doi.org/10.1016/0167-4870(93)90004-5

Trönnberg, C. C., & Hemlin, S. (2012). Banker's lending decision making: A psychological approach. *Managerial Finance*. https://doi.org/10.1108/03074351211266775

Wang, X., Xu, Y. C., Lu, T., & Zhang, C. (2020). Why do borrowers default on online loans? An inquiry of their psychology mechanism. *Internet Research, 30*(4), 1203–1228. https://doi.org/10.1108/INTR-05-2019-0183

Webley, P., & Nyhus, E. K. (2001). Life-cycle and dispositional routes into problem debt. *British Journal of Psychology, 92*(3), 423–446. https://doi.org/10.1348/000712601162275

Weiss, R. S. (2006). The attachment bond in childhood and adulthood. In *Attachment across the life cycle* (pp. 74–84). Routledge.

Wilson, F., Carter, S., Tagg, S., Shaw, E., & Lam, W. (2007). Bank loan officers' perceptions of business owners: The role of gender. *British Journal of Management, 18*(2), 154–171. https://doi.org/10.1111/j.1467-8551.2006.00508.x

Worthy, S. L., Jonkman, J., & Blinn-Pike, L. (2010). Sensation-seeking, risk-taking, and problematic financial behaviors of college students. *Journal of Family and Economic Issues, 31*(2), 161–170. https://doi.org/10.1007/s10834-010-9183-6

Zuckerman, M. (1979). Beyond the optimal level of arousal. *Hillsdale, NJ: Lawrence Erlbraum Associates.*

Zuckerman, M., & Kuhlman, D. M. (2000). Personality and risk-taking: Common biosocial factors. *Journal of Personality, 68*(6), 999–1029. https://doi.org/10.1111/1467-6494.00124

Online Learning and University Students' Anxiety During the Covid-19 Pandemic

Serveh Sharifi Far and Thomas E. Hunt

Abstract This study explored anxiety among students studying online during the Covid-19 pandemic. Fifty university students on a statistical methodology course in a UK university completed a survey assessing anxiety pertaining to online learning, mathematics, computers, state-trait, and the pandemic situation. Online learning anxiety (OLA) was positively and significantly related to the other forms of anxiety. Women reported significantly higher OLA compared to men before controlling for other types of anxiety. After controlling for gender and other anxieties, computer anxiety remained a significant predictor of OLA, suggesting support may be best directed towards the use of computers and possibly the use of technology more broadly. Self-reports also revealed a range of triggers of anxiety, including worry concerning online distraction. These findings offer insight into ways in which educators can support students in an online learning context.

Keywords Computer anxiety · Higher education · Mathematics anxiety · Student wellbeing · Online teaching

1 Introduction

Higher education was affected by the onset of the Covid-19 pandemic and required a change of operational mode from the usual in-person education to a mostly or fully online mode (see, for example, Crawford et al., 2020; Johnson et al., 2020). Such a rapid change introduced challenges in communication for both educators and students and required an increased use of digital applications. Online education has also offered flexibility in time, location, and costs as an alternative to face-to-face learning and teaching.

S. Sharifi Far (✉)
School of Mathematics, University of Edinburgh, Edinburgh, UK
e-mail: serveh.sharifi@ed.ac.uk

T. E. Hunt
School of Psychology, University of Derby, Derby, UK
e-mail: t.hunt@derby.ac.uk

P. Macaulay and L. Tan (eds.), *Applied Psychology Readings*,
https://doi.org/10.1007/978-981-99-2613-8_4

Despite the obvious benefits that an online learning approach has presented in response to the recent pandemic, several immediate challenges have been identified, e.g. reduced social interaction and feelings of isolation (Almendingen et al., 2021), technical issues and internet access (Adnan & Anwar, 2020), distractions and uncertainty about assessments (Idris et al., 2021), and difficulties maintaining focus (Asgari et al., 2021). The Office for National Statistics conducted research into the impact of the Covid-19 pandemic on the behaviour and well-being of students in higher education in England from September to December 2020, including the Student Covid Insights Survey (SCIS). According to the SCIS, compared to the general population, students reported lower levels of life satisfaction and happiness, as well as higher levels of anxiety. It also showed that over half of students reported a detrimental impact of the pandemic on their mental health and well-being (Office for National Statistics, 2020). Other recent work has supported this finding, with over 90% of undergraduates in their sample reporting studying online during the Covid-19 outbreak as either stressful or very stressful (Oducado & Estoque, 2021), and others showing that over one-fifth of university students experienced severe or extremely severe anxiety during the recent pandemic (Jiang et al., 2021).

The present study focused on university students' feelings of anxiety related to online learning on a specific course and how it was related to a range of other anxieties, including mathematics, computer, state-trait, and the pandemic situation. We asked students about the main triggers of online learning anxiety (OLA) and investigated whether it was significantly different according to their engagement in the course and various demographic and course properties.

2 Theoretical Framework

2.1 Anxiety and Online Learning

Online learning has been a focus of education research in the past two decades and has been defined in various terms. One broad definition is "the use of the internet in some way to enhance the interaction between teacher and student" which covers both asynchronous and synchronous forms of interaction (Curtain, 2002). The most common synonymous terms used to define online learning are, "e-learning", "blended-learning", "online education/course", "distance education/learning", and "web-based Learning". The different definitions usually include some common terms including, "technology", "interactivity", and "time- asynchronous and synchronous" (Singh & Thurman, 2019).

Online learning can be a source of anxiety for students due to the unfamiliar nature of the learning environment, lack of clear guidelines, technical difficulties, and limited contact with other parties involved (Abdous, 2019). Understanding the pattern and sources of such feelings can be crucial for instructors regarding course design and interaction with students.

Bolliger and Halupa (2012) developed a course anxiety scale with 18 items and three elements: computer, the internet, and the online course. Among a cohort of students in an online doctoral programme, they found that anxiety levels were relatively moderate and did not significantly change over time. However, the sample included students studying at a high level of education, potentially representing greater familiarity and competence with computers, the internet, and online courses. Hilliard (2017) explored undergraduate students' perceptions and experiences of anxiety in an online collaborative project using a combination of online surveys and interviews. They concluded that anxiety was common among respondents, it gradually decreased throughout the project, and was mainly associated with the uncertainty involved in such frameworks. Abdous (2019) studied the influence of orientation satisfaction and the sense of preparedness for an online course on students' feelings of anxiety. They measured OLA (with a binary yes/no response) using a question of whether taking an online course had increased participants' feelings of anxiety. Their findings showed that female, full-time, and first-year online students had higher anxiety. Further to this, greater prior online learning experience and the sense of preparedness were factors associated with lower feelings of anxiety.

In this study, we investigated several demographic variables and factors related to the course design to realise how they relate to OLA. However, it is important to understand how other forms of anxiety contribute to students' OLA, namely computer anxiety and state-trait anxiety. Due to the nature of the course and the unusual situation at the time, we also included measures of mathematics anxiety and anxiety associated with the Covid-19 pandemic.

2.2 *Other Anxieties (Computer, Mathematics, State-Trait, Covid-19 Pandemic Situation)*

Computer anxiety is different from negative attitudes towards computers and comprises feelings of fear, apprehension, intimidation, hostility, and worry associated with using computers, which is further related to resistance and avoidance (Heinssen et al., 1987). Different scales have been constructed to measure computer anxiety, including the Computer Anxiety Rating Scale (CARS) by Heinssen et al. (1987) and the adaptation by Bolliger and Halupa (2012). As part of an overall measure of online cooperative learning anxiety, Yoshida et al. (2016) identified a computer anxiety subscale, which correlated ($r = 0.58$) with the online learning anxiety subscale. Thus, whilst related to OLA, computer anxiety may be considered a unique construct.

Mathematics (maths) anxiety is defined as "feelings of tension and anxiety that interfere with the manipulation of numbers and the solving of mathematical problems in a wide variety of ordinary life and academic situations" (Richardson & Suinn, 1972, p.551). There are several published self-report measures of maths anxiety, including the Abbreviated Math Anxiety Scale (Hopko et al., 2003), which includes nine items and two factors of maths learning and maths evaluation anxiety. Previous research has shown that maths anxiety is related to maths avoidance (Ahmed, 2018; Chipman et al., 2002) and poorer maths performance (Barroso et al., 2021; Zhang et al., 2019). Given that our study involved students enrolled in a course with mathematical content, it was important that maths anxiety was measured in the context of a switch to online learning.

General anxiety is separable into two types: state anxiety, which is a temporary reaction to specific adverse events or situations, and trait anxiety, which is a more stable personality feature and is related to a tendency to respond to various situations with concerns, troubles and worries (Saviola et al., 2020). The Spielberger State-Trait Anxiety Inventory (STAI) is frequently used to measure these two aspects of human anxiety and has been translated to several languages. Zsido et al. (2020) provide a short and reliable version of this scale as a practical option where it is not feasible to use the full version. The inclusion of a measure of general anxiety is useful when assessing the extent to which related, domain-specific, anxieties account for unique variance in a specified outcome variable over and above general anxiety. Conceptually, evidence of divergence is important when variables are interrelated, e.g. in the case of maths anxiety-computer anxiety (Birenbaum & Eylath, 1994), computer anxiety-general trait anxiety (Gaudron & Vignoli, 2022), and general trait anxiety-maths anxiety (Batashvili et al., 2022).

The Covid-19 pandemic was the reason for a rapid switch to online teaching and it also affected many people's personal lives. It is reasonable to expect it to be related to other types of anxieties and to influence students' experience of online learning. As data in the current study were collected in the early stages of the pandemic, we opted to include a single-item measure to capture self-reported increases in anxiety associated with the Covid-19 situation at the time.

2.3 *Purpose of Study*

The purpose of this study was to investigate university students' feelings of anxiety in relation to taking a specific course after the format of study was changed from the usual in-person, on-campus form to online due to the Covid-19 pandemic. The research questions to answer are:

(1) To what extent are students anxious about online learning during the Covid-19 pandemic?
(2) What are the main triggers of OLA during the pandemic?
(3) How is OLA related to other relevant types of anxiety?
(4) How do engagement in the course, prior experience in online learning, and demographic factors relate to OLA?

3 Methods

3.1 Sample and Procedure

The study was conducted in the School of Mathematics, University of Edinburgh, U.K. in semester one (Autumn) of the 2020–21 academic year, which was the first semester of online/hybrid teaching due to the Covid-19 pandemic. The online, anonymous survey (on www.onlinesurveys.ac.uk) was advertised to all (239) students who took a 10-credit course in Statistical Methodology. Of those, 50 students (21%) completed the survey. The sample comprised an equal number of men (49%) and women (49%) and one participant (2%) preferred not to report their gender. The majority of participants (63%) were in the age category 21–25 years, 29% were 17–20 years, and 8% were 26–30 years. Most (59%) participants were undergraduates and 57% of participants reported that English is their native language. 71% of these students had signed up for only the online tutorials and 29% for only the on-campus tutorials. Students were asked "Where do you usually use a computer to access this online course's material?", 84% chose "a personal space", 12% chose "a shared space", and 4% chose "a study space at the university". Of participants, 90% did not have a job and 10% had a part-time job, whilst 83% stated that they had not taken any online course prior to the academic year 2020–21.

The course is compulsory for third-year undergraduate students in the Mathematics and Statistics programme and optional for other undergraduates and postgraduate students. The course ran as a hybrid course with pre-recorded lectures, digital quizzes and assessments, tutorials in a workshop style with online and on-campus options, online programming exercises, online synchronous office hours, and an anonymous text-based support forum. With the exception of an option for in-person on-campus tutorials (which 29% of the class signed up for), all other activities were held online. Therefore, we refer to the course as an online course in this manuscript. The course assessment comprised 30% coursework and 70% final exam.

3.2 Measures

Online learning anxiety. Online learning anxiety was measured using a six-item scale, in which responses can range from 1 (strongly disagree) to 5 (strongly agree), slightly adjusted from the items used by Bolliger and Halupa (2012). Ten possible triggers of anxiety in online teaching and learning, slightly adjusted from Abdous (2019), were presented to students in a table to indicate which ones were relevant to them.

Computer anxiety. Computer anxiety was measured using a six-item scale, with response options ranging from 1 (strongly disagree) to 5 (strongly agree), taken from Bolliger and Halupa (2012).

Mathematics anxiety. The Abbreviated Mathematics Anxiety Scale (AMAS; Hopko et al., 2003) is a nine-item scale in which participants are required to respond to how anxious they feel in a range of mathematical contexts. We used the AMAS items with a slight change in the instructions and response options. In order to assess participants' self-reported maths anxiety that is typical for them during normal, i.e. face-to-face learning, we changed the instructions to "While taking an on-campus mathematical course (for example in the previous academic year), the following situations make me anxious". Consequently, we adjusted the response format to 1 (strongly disagree) to 5 (strongly agree).

State and trait anxiety. State and trait anxiety were measured using the short version of the Spielberger State-Trait Anxiety Inventory, reported by Zsido et al. (2020). Five items pertained to how participants feel "right now" (state) and five pertained to how they feel "generally" (trait). The response options range from 1 (not at all) to 4 (very much so).

Anxiety related to the Covid-19 pandemic. As a brief measure of whether participants felt the Covid-19 pandemic had increased any feelings of anxiety, we asked the following question: "Has the current situation related to Covid-19 (self-isolation, quarantine, ...) increased your feelings of anxiety?" The response options ranged from 1 (not at all) to 4 (very much so).

Engagement. As per the approach used by Dixon (2010), engagement was measured by asking students which course activities they find engaging and how they rate their engagement in the course on a scale of 1 (not engaged) to 4 (very engaged).

The instrument also included six demographic questions on gender, age group, study level, type of study space, employment status, and whether English was a native language. Other questions related to the course included whether participants took online or on-campus tutorials and whether they had taken online courses prior to this academic year to factor in their experience in online teaching and learning.

3.3 Data Analyses

There were a small number of missing values and a list-wise deletion method was used in each statistical test or model. Descriptive statistics and frequencies were calculated for demographic and course-related variables. Descriptive statistics and bivariate correlations between the different forms of anxiety were also generated. Then, the bivariate correlation between engagement in the course and OLA was calculated.

Independent samples t-tests and one-way ANOVAs were applied to test the effects of demographic and course-related categorical variables on OLA. The assumptions of equal variances and normality were checked and, depending on the result, the appropriate variations of the tests were used. Three normal linear regression models were fitted to examine (i) the relationship between OLA and the demographic and course-related categorical predictors which were found to be significant in the preceding tests; (ii) the relationship between the OLA and the other types of anxiety; and (iii) the effect of all the predictors on OLA in one model.

4 Results

4.1 Descriptive Statistics

In reporting their overall engagement level in the course, 6% of students were "very engaged", 44% "engaged", 42% "somewhat engaged", and 8% "not engaged". Out of the eight different course activities named in the questionnaire, students chose the following as the most engaging ones: digital weekly quizzes (78%), digital biweekly assessments (71%), pre-recorded lectures (59%), text-based support forum (47%), and tutorial sessions (47%). The other activities were extra exercises (37%), programming tasks on the cloud (25%), and online synchronous office hours (10%).

Six types of anxiety. The descriptive statistics for the six types of anxiety are summarised in Table 1.

Data for each type of anxiety were tested for normality using the Shapiro–Wilk test at the 5% significance level. State Anxiety and Covid-19 Anxiety did not pass the normality test ($p < 0.01$).

Bivariate Pearson correlations between the anxiety variables are presented in Table 2. All types of anxiety were significantly and positively correlated and OLA was moderately-to-strongly related to all other forms of anxiety.

Triggers of anxiety in online learning. The frequencies of self-reported triggers associated with OLA are reported in Table 3.

Online learning anxiety and engagement in the course. A Pearson's correlation test showed no significant relationship between OLA and self-reported engagement in the course, $r(48) = -0.21, p = 0.15$.

Table 1 Summary statistics of observations for the investigated anxiety variables

Anxiety measure	Range	Median	Mean	SD	Item mean	Cronbach's alpha
Online Learning Anxiety	7–29	18	17.82	5.07	2.97	0.79
Mathematics Anxiety	9–39	28	27.37	6.03	3.04	0.86
Computer Anxiety	6–25	14	13.94	4.49	2.32	0.87
State Anxiety	5–19	8.5	9.38	3.38	1.88	0.77
Trait Anxiety	6–20	12	12.32	3.80	2.46	0.79
Covid-19 Anxiety	1–4	2	2.44	1.01	2.44	N/A

Table 2 Bivariate Pearson correlations between the investigated anxiety variables

	(1)	(2)	(3)	(4)	(5)	(6)
Online learning anxiety (1)	1	0.41**	0.50**	0.36**	0.49**	0.39**
Mathematics anxiety (2)		1	0.25	0.40**	0.44**	0.30*
Computer anxiety (3)			1	0.26	0.33*	0.35*
State anxiety (4)				1	0.39**	0.31*
Trait anxiety (5)					1	0.56**
Covid-19 anxiety (6)						1

** $p < 0.01$, * $p < 0.05$

Table 3 Percentage of factors triggering anxiety in the online course

Item	Percentages (counts)
Risk of online distraction—for example, wasting time on social media	54% (26)
Not having enough immediate classroom interaction with faculty and students	52% (25)
Having to ask questions in online tutorials	50% (24)
Not having enough clear explanations on what to do	50% (24)
Lack of physical classroom environment	40% (19)
Not having enough interaction with classmates	40% (19)
Not having enough face-to-face time with faculty	31% (15)
Not having enough feedback from faculty	27% (13)
Technical difficulties	25% (12)
Having to ask questions on the online text-based forum	25% (12)
Other	10% (5)

Testing group differences in online learning anxiety. Independent samples t-tests were conducted to test if OLA differed according to programme level (UG/PG), having a job (no job/part-time), if English was the participant's native language (yes/no), tutorial format (online/on-campus), and whether they had taken online courses before (yes/no). No significant differences were observed (all $p > 0.2$). However, women (mean = 20.00) reported significantly higher OLA than men (mean = 15.88), $t(46) = 3.01, p < 0.01, d = 0.87$.

A one-way independent measures ANOVA with equal variances showed no significant difference in OLA between age groups, $F(2, 46) = 0.25, p = 0.78$. For the study space variable, the category "university provided space" had only two observations, thus a non-parametric, Kruskal–Wallis test was conducted, which demonstrated no significant effect, $H(2) = 5.17, p = 0.08$.

4.2 Modelling Online Learning Anxiety

Using Normal Linear Regression, we examined the relationship between OLA (the outcome variable) and gender, the predictor variable that was found to be significant in the preceding tests (Model 1). Next, we examined the relationship between OLA and the other types of anxiety as predictors (Model 2). Then we fitted a normal linear regression with both sets of the previously included predictors (Model 3). The model assumptions were checked for all three models (collinearity of the predictors, normality and constant variance of the residuals) and no deviations were detected. The model parameter estimates, standard errors, and p-values are given in Table 4.

Model 1 showed that gender was a significant predictor of OLA, such that women reported higher OLA than men. Model 2 demonstrated that computer anxiety was the only form of anxiety that was significantly related to OLA, whereby a higher level of computer anxiety was associated with a higher level of OLA. Model 3 combined both sets of predictors and showed that computer anxiety remained a significant predictor of OLA, whereas gender did not.

Table 4 Normal linear regression models predicting online learning anxiety

Predictors	Model 1			Model 2			Model 3		
	Est	SE	P	Est	SE	P	Est	SE	p
Intercept	15.875	0.970	<0.01**	2.401	3.097	0.443	1.820	3.618	0.618
Gender (woman)	4.125	1.372	<0.01**				−0.524	1.637	0.751
Maths anxiety				0.148	0.115	0.204	0.159	0.121	0.196
Computer anxiety				0.405	0.145	<0.01**	0.429	0.165	0.013*
State anxiety				0.105	0.205	0.611	0.113	0.208	0.590
Trait anxiety				0.332	0.210	0.121	0.337	0.213	0.121
Covid-19 anxiety				0.318	0.723	0.662	0.343	0.735	0.643
	Adjusted $R^2 = 0.15$ $F(1,46) = 9.04$, $p = 0.004$			Adjusted $R^2 = 0.36$ $F(5, 42) = 6.26$, $p < 0.001$			Adjusted $R^2 = 0.34$ $F(6, 41) = 5.12$, $p < 0.001$		

** $p < 0.01$, * $p < 0.05$

5 Discussion

We aimed to assess the extent to which OLA, as reported during a global pandemic, relates to other forms of anxiety and a range of demographic variables. In answer to our first research question, data for OLA were normally distributed. Reassuringly, the mean of OLA was reasonably low. However, several students indicated a moderate or high level of OLA. Moreover, in response to the direct question of whether taking the current online course had increased feelings of anxiety, 42% said yes. This is congruent with findings that general anxiety (Wang et al., 2020) and stress associated with online learning (Oducado & Estoque, 2021) increased during the Covid-19 pandemic, with some research suggesting that OLA does not necessarily wain as a result of experience (Unger & Meiran, 2020). Oducado and Estoque (2021) noted that over 85% of their sample of undergraduates found it more difficult to focus during online learning. This further tallies with other work, showing that very few students who temporarily switched to online learning during the pandemic wanted online learning to continue (Jojoa et al., 2021).

In answering the second research question, self-reports in the current study suggested multiple triggers of OLA, with the risk of online distraction, e.g. wasting time on social media, being the most frequently cited trigger of OLA. This is worth noting since it is the only trigger (out of the 10 listed), other than "technical difficulties", that is not explicitly related to course features. Consequently, educators may need to consider ways of supporting students regarding online distractions. Conversely, it is important to note cases where perceived benefits of online learning have been reported. For example, Lemay et al. (2021) found that the majority of students sampled reported being better able to focus on lectures online without the distraction of other people. However, their sample included pre-university students who may not have experienced the many challenges faced by university students living away from home; students who resided with their families during the Covid-19 lockdown experienced a more "painless" adaptation to distance learning (Demetriou et al., 2021).

Investigating the third research question showed that all of the anxieties measured were interrelated. Online learning anxiety was positively and significantly correlated with all other types of anxiety. It had the strongest correlations with computer and trait anxiety which indicates that participants who are anxious about using computers and those who are generally anxious reported greater OLA. Results further showed that a significant and positive relationship between computer anxiety and OLA was present even after controlling for all other variables in the model, including multiple anxieties. This finding chimes with previous work that has demonstrated the importance of computer anxiety in the context of OLA (Yoshida et al., 2016). This highlights the need to target computer anxiety as a potential strategy for addressing OLA more generally. Indeed, a key component of this may include computer self-efficacy, supported by the previous finding that computer self-efficacy plays a significant role in mediating the impact of anxiety on perceived ease of use among university students (Saade & Kira, 2009). Thus, one possible solution would be to provide all students with more computer-based training and technical support during the online learning process. Such support may also need to expand to the broader online learning environment, given that a more straightforward adaptation to distance learning methods has been associated with fewer stress symptoms (Demetriou et al., 2021). Also, it is important to note that support infers that students have no internet access issues, which may not be the case in under-developed countries (Adnan & Anwar, 2020). Relatedly, it may also be necessary to prepare students for online learning in advance of any engagement as a way of mitigating potential anxiety (Riaz et al., 2021).

The importance of computer anxiety in the context of OLA also raises an important conceptual point regarding the nature of OLA and whether computer anxiety should be considered a component of OLA or whether it is a distinct construct. Items on measures of computer anxiety, such as the one used in the present study, relate explicitly to computers rather than specific forms of technology, e.g. smartphones or tablets, e.g. "I am apprehensive about working on computers" or "I avoid working on computers". As such, the term "computers" may be viewed in a rather nuanced way and perhaps ignores the myriad technology now used to facilitate online learning, including hybrid technology and the high frequency of learners who access online classes via a smartphone (Saha et al., 2021). Whilst, computers may be considered an integral part of online learning, the nature of online learning today means that students can engage with multiple technologies. In addition, engaging in an in-person course does not preclude students from using computers. Indeed, in a world that increasingly values computer-based skills, it is possible that computers are becoming less suitable as a way of distinguishing between in-person and online learning. As such, others (e.g. Yoshida et al., 2016) have introduced the term "technology-related anxiety" as an alternative to computer anxiety. Interestingly, however, a series of ad hoc semi-partial correlations in the current study showed no significant relationship between computer anxiety and each of the other anxieties after controlling for OLA (all $p > 0.25$). This additional finding suggests that computer anxiety does not contribute unique variance in trait, state, and maths anxiety once its relation with OLA is controlled for.

In answer to our fourth research question, an analysis of group differences demonstrated that women reported significantly higher OLA than men, showing a large effect size. This is consistent with recent findings in which female university students have reported significantly greater OLA than males (Abdous, 2019; Riquelme et al., 2021). Whilst this finding is typical of gender differences in general anxiety and maths anxiety (e.g. Batashvili et al., 2022), it highlights the need to understand why women reported greater OLA than men and how this may then inform strategies to support female students. Testing of other group differences in the present study revealed no significant effects.

Some limitations of the current study should be noted. The sample comprised students from only one course from one university, which limits generalisability. Given that students were enrolled in a statistical methodology course, they required a good background in mathematics, therefore increasing the homogeneity of the sample. Nevertheless, despite having similar educational backgrounds, little skew was present in the data, with OLA values demonstrating a close-to-normal distribution. Also, all participants were 30 years or younger; other work has found that OLA varies as a function of generation, with older participants reporting higher OLA (Elshami et al., 2021). In addition, a larger sample size would facilitate the testing of more complex models that incorporate more fully the interrelations between the range of anxieties measured. Finally, the cross-sectional nature of the current study means that causal inferences cannot be made concerning the specific impact of the Covid-19 pandemic on OLA; for example, some research has shown online learning anxiety existed pre-Covid-19 (Kira et al., 2018). However, others have found general anxiety to increase following a move to online learning (Wang et al., 2020), along with a positive correlation between satisfaction with online learning and general anxiety during the Covid-19 pandemic (Fawaz & Samaha, 2020). Also, a large proportion of the current sample retrospectively reported an increase in anxiety since the start of the Covid-19 pandemic.

In conclusion, in a sample of university students who unexpectedly found themselves learning online during the Covid-19 pandemic, many reported increased levels of anxiety, with women reporting considerably higher OLA than men. After controlling for gender and other forms of anxiety, computer anxiety remained a significant predictor of OLA, suggesting support may be best directed towards the use of computers and possibly the use of technology more broadly. Results revealed a range of self-reported triggers of anxiety, including worry concerning online distraction. This highlights an aspect of computer—or technology—anxiety that may be more prominent than previously expected. Other triggers included interactions in an online environment, but also the general absence of interaction with students and staff in a physical learning environment. These findings offer insight into ways in which educators can support students in an online learning context.

Acknowledgements We would like to thank Chris Sangwin and Steven O'Hagan at the School of Mathematics, the University of Edinburgh for helpful discussions on early stages of this work. We also gratefully acknowledge the contribution of the research participants.

References

Abdous, M. (2019). Influence of satisfaction and preparedness on online students' feelings of anxiety. *The Internet and Higher Education, 41*, 34–44. https://doi.org/10.1016/j.iheduc.2019.01.001

Adnan, M., & Anwar, K. (2020). Online learning amid the COVID-19 pandemic: Students' perspectives. *Journal of Pedagogical Sociology and Psychology, 2*(1), 45–51. https://doi.org/10.33902/JPSP. 2020261309

Ahmed, W. (2018). Developmental trajectories of math anxiety during adolescence: Associations with STEM career choice. *Journal of Adolescence, 67*, 158–166. https://doi.org/10.1016/j.adolescence.2018.06.010

Almendingen, K., Morseth, M. S., Gjølstad, E., Brevik, A., & Tørris, C. (2021). Student's experiences with online teaching following COVID-19 lockdown: A mixed methods explorative study. *PLoS ONE, 16*(8), e0250378. https://doi.org/10.1371/journal.pone.0250378

Asgari, S., Trajkovic, J., Rahmani, M., Zhang, W., Lo, R. C., & Sciortino, A. (2021). An observational study of engineering online education during the COVID-19 pandemic. *PLoS ONE, 16*(4), e0250041. https://doi.org/10.1371/journal.pone.0250041

Barroso, C., Ganley, C. M., McGraw, A. L., Geer, E. A., Hart, S. A., & Daucourt, M. C. (2021). A meta-analysis of the relation between math anxiety and math achievement. *Psychological Bulletin, 147*, 134–168. https://doi.org/10.1037/bul0000307

Batashvili, M., Cipora, K., & Hunt, T. E. (2022). Measurement of mathematics anxiety in an Israeli adult population. *Journal of Numerical Cognition, 8*(1), 148–165. https://doi.org/10.5964/jnc.6531

Birenbaum, M., & Eylath, S. (1994). Who is afraid of statistics? Correlates of statistics anxiety among students of educational sciences. *Educational Research, 36*(1), 93–98. https://doi.org/10.1080/0013188940360110

Bolliger, D. U., & Halupa, C. (2012). Student perceptions of satisfaction and anxiety in an online doctoral program. *Distance Education, 33*(1), 81–98. https://doi.org/10.1080/01587919.2012.667961

Chipman, S., Krantz, D., & Silver, R. (1992). Mathematics anxiety and science careers among able college students. *Psychological Science, 3*, 292–295.

Crawford, J., Butler-Henderson, K., Rudolph, J., Malkawi, B., Burton, R., Magni, P. A., & Lam, S. (2020). COVID-19: 20 countries' higher education intra-period digital pedagogy responses. *Journal of Applied Learning & Teaching, 3*(1), 1–28. https://doi.org/10.37074/jalt.2020.3.1.7

Curtain, R. (2002). Online delivery in the vocational education and training sector: Improving cost effectiveness. *National Centre for Vocational Education Research.* https://www.ncver.edu.au/research-and-statistics/publications/all-publications/online-delivery-in-the-vocational-education-and-training-sector-improving-cost-effectiveness.

Demetriou, L., Keramioti, L., & Hadjicharalambous, D. (2021). Examining the relationship between distance learning processes and university students' anxiety in times of Covid-19. *European Journal of Social Sciences Studies, 6*(2), 123–141. https://doi.org/10.46827/ejsss.v6i2.1012

Dixon, M. D. (2010). Creating effective student engagement in online courses: What do students find engaging? *Journal of the Scholarship of Teaching and Learning, 10*(2), 1–13.

Elshami, W., Saravanan, C., Taha, M. H., Abdalla, M. E., Abuzaid, M., & Al Kawas, S. (2021). Bridging the gap in online learning anxiety among different generations in health professions education. *SQU Medical Journal, 21*(4), 539–548. https://doi.org/10.18295/squmj.4.2021.040

Fawaz, M., & Samaha, A. (2021). E-learning: Depression, anxiety, and stress symptomatology among Lebanese university students during COVID-19 quarantine. *Nursing Forum, 56*, 52–57. https://doi.org/10.1111/nuf.12521

Gaudron, J.-P., & Vignoli, E. (2002). Assessing computer anxiety with the interaction model of anxiety: Development and validation of the computer anxiety trait subscale. *Computers in Human Behavior, 18*, 315–325. https://doi.org/10.1016/S0747-5632(01)00039-5

Heinssen, R. K., Glass, C. R., & Knight, L. A. (1987). Assessing computer anxiety: Development and validation of the computer anxiety rating scale. *Computers in Human Behavior, 3*(1), 49–59. https://doi.org/10.1016/0747-5632(87)90010-0

Hilliard, J. (2017). Students' perceptions and experiences of anxiety in an online collaborative project. *MRes thesis The Open University.* https://doi.org/10.21954/ou.ro.0000cd42

Hopko, D. R., Mahadevan, R., Bare, R. L., & Hunt, M. K. (2003). The abbreviated math anxiety scale (AMAS): Construction, validity, and reliability. *Assessment, 10*(2), 178–182. https://doi.org/10.1177/1073191103010002008

Idris, F., Zulkipli, I. N., Abdul-Mumin, K. H., Ahmad, S. R., Mitha, S., Rahman, H. A., Rajabalaya, R., David, S. R., & Naing, L. (2021). Academic experiences, physical and mental health impact of COVID-19 pandemic on students and lecturers in health care education. *BMC Medical Education, 21*, 542. https://doi.org/10.1186/s12909-021-02968-2

Jiang, N., Yan-Li, S., Pamanee, K., & Sriyanto, J. (2021). Depression, anxiety, and stress during the COVID-19 pandemic: Comparison among higher education students in four countries in the Asia-Pacific region. *Journal of Population and Social Studies, 29*, 370–383. http://doi.org/https://doi.org/10.25133/JPSSv292021.023

Johnson, N., Veletsianos, G., & Seaman, J. (2020). US Faculty and administrators' experiences and approaches in the early weeks of the COVID-19 pandemic. *Online Learning, 24*(2), 6–21.

Jojoa, M., Lazaro, E., Garcia-Zapirain, B., Gonzalez, M. J., & Urizar, E. (2021). The impact of COVID 19 on university staff and students from Iberoamerica: Online learning and teaching experience. *International Journal of Environmental Research Public Health, 18*, 5820. https://doi.org/10.3390/ijerph18115820

Kira, D, Nebebe, F. & Saadé, R. G. (2018). The persistence of anxiety experienced by new generation in online learning. In *Proceedings of the Informing Science and Information Technology Education Conference, La Vearne, California* (pp. 79–88). Santa Rosa, CA: Informing Science Institute. https://doi.org/10.28945/4040

Lemay, D. J., Bazelais, P., & Doleck, T. (2021). Transition to online learning during the COVID-19 pandemic. *Computers in Human Behavior Reports, 4*, 100130. https://doi.org/10.1016/j.chbr.2021.100130

Oducado, R. M. & Estoque, H. (2021). Online learning in nursing education during the COVID-19 pandemic: Stress, satisfaction, and academic performance. *Journal of Nursing Practice, 4*(2), 143–153. http://dx.doi.org/https://doi.org/10.30994/jnp.v4i2.128

Office for National Statistics. (2020). Coronavirus and the impact on students in higher education in England: September to December 2020, https://www.ons.gov.uk/peoplepopulationandcommunity/educationandchildcare/articles/coronavirusandtheimpactonstudentsinhighereducationinenglandseptembertodecember2020/2020-12-21

Riaz, H., Tahir, W., Irfan, S., Saeed, W. & Khizar, U. (2021). Readiness for online learning as a predictor of academic stress and anxiety. *iRAD Journal of Management, 3*(2), 146–155. https://doi.org/10.52131/jom.2021.0302.0034

Richardson, F. C., & Suinn, R. M. (1972). The mathematics anxiety rating scale: Psychometric data. *Journal of Counselling Psychology, 19*(6), 551–554. https://doi.org/10.1037/h0033456

Riquelme, V., Maureira, N. C., Navarro, C. V., & Puente, C. T. (2021). Ansiedad al aprendizaje en línea: relación con actitud, género, entorno y salud mental en universitarios. *Revista Digital de Investigación en Docencia Universitaria, 15*(1), E1284. https://doi.org/10.19083/ridu.2021.1284

Saadé, R. G., & Kira, D. (2009). Computer anxiety in e-learning: The effect of computer self-efficacy. *Journal of Information Technology Education: Research, 8*(1), 177–191. https://doi.org/10.28945/166

Saha, A., Dutta, A., & Sifat, R. I. (2021). The mental impact of digital divide due to COVID-19 pandemic induced emergency online learning at undergraduate level: Evidence from undergraduate students from Dhaka City. *Journal of Affective Disorders, 294*, 170–179. https://doi.org/10.1016/j.jad.2021.07.045

Saviola, F., Pappaianni, E., Monti, A., Grecucci, A., Jovicich, J., & De Pisapia, N. (2020). Trait and state anxiety are mapped differently in the human brain. ***Scientific Reports, 10***, 11112. https://doi.org/10.1038/s41598-020-68008-z

Singh, V., & Thurman, A. (2019). How many ways can we define online learning? A systematic literature review of definitions of online learning (1988–2018). *American Journal of Distance Education, 33*(4), 289–306. https://doi.org/10.1080/08923647.2019.1663082

Unger, S., & Meiran, W. R. (2020). Student attitudes towards online education during the COVID-19 viral outbreak of 2020: Distance learning in a time of social distance. *International Journal of Technology in Education and Science (IJTES), 4*(4), 256–266. https://doi.org/10.46328/ijtes.v4i4.107

Wang, C., Zhao, H., & Zhang, H. (2020). Chinese college students have higher anxiety in new semester of online learning during COVID-19: A machine learning approach. *Frontiers in Psychology, 11*, 587413. https://doi.org/10.3389/fpsyg.2020.587413

Yoshida, H., Tani, S., Uchida, T., Masui, J., Fukushima, M., & Nakayama, A. (2016). Development and validation of the online cooperative learning anxiety scale. *International Journal of Information and Education Technology, 6*(5), 357–364. https://doi.org/10.7763/IJIET.2016.V6.714

Zhang, J., Zhao, N., & Kong, Q. P. (2019). The relationship between math anxiety and math performance: A meta-analytic investigation. *Frontiers in Psychology, 10*, 1613–1613. https://doi.org/10.3389/fpsyg.2019.01613

Zsido, A. N., Teleki, S. A., Csokasi, K., Rozsa, S., & Bandi, S. A. (2020). Development of the short version of the Spielberger state-trait anxiety inventory. *Psychiatry Research, 291*, 113–223. https://doi.org/10.1016/j.psychres.2020.113223

Psychological Well-Being in Highly Sensitive People

Regina V. Ershova

Abstract (Aron and Aron, Journal of Personality and Social Psychology 73:345–368, 1997) developed a personality construct of high sensitivity, characterized by a physiologically predetermined sensory processing sensitivity. Their unidimensional scale, the Highly Sensitive Person Scale (HSPS), measures the level of sensory processing sensitivity and can predict the negative emotional, social, behavioral outcomes such as social phobia, anxiety, depression, low self-efficacy, etc. However, previous research questioned the nature of the HSPS questionnaire, and proposed its division into two- or three-factor models. In a large body of studies SPS is seen as a trait that influences a life satisfaction of a person, but there is no clear evidence about the relationship of SPS with psychological well-being. Two studies (N = 860) extended previous findings in terms of the inner structure of sensory processing sensitivity and its connection with life outcomes. The objective of the study was to give the first evidence of the Highly Sensitive Person Scale's psychometric properties in a Russian-speaking population alongside the Aron and Aron scale and to describe the relations of sensitivity with the Psychological Well-being Scale (Riff, 1989). A sample of 860 respondents participated in the study: 350 undergraduate university student volunteers and 510 social media users (613 females and 247 males aged 15–43, M age = 20.8, SD age = 3.5). They filled out two questionnaires. Results did not confirm the initial linear model nor the three-factor solution. The hierarchical cluster and confirmatory analyses suggest that sensory processing sensitivity (SPS) can be described in a two-factor model consisting of 'Ease of Excitation' and 'Low Sensory Threshold' subscales. The t-test showed that only one subscale of Psychological well-being (personal growth) is disconnected with high sensitivity. Highly sensitive individuals are characterized by difficulties in relationships with others, limited number of interpersonal contacts, dependence on opinions and assessments of others, conformity, and low self-esteem therefore high sensitivity may be seen as a factor of psychological well-being decrease. Future studies should expand research on SPS as a sensitivity marker to both positive and negative outcomes, more research

R. V. Ershova (✉)
Department of Psychology and Pedagogy, Russian Friendship University, Moscow, Russia
e-mail: ershova-rv@rudn.ru

Department of Psychology, State University of Humanities and Social Studies, Moscow, Russia

P. Macaulay and L. Tan (eds.), *Applied Psychology Readings*,
https://doi.org/10.1007/978-981-99-2613-8_5

is needed that manipulates the positive or negative impact of SPS on life satisfaction and well-being and the study of dynamic changes in SPS in connection to psychological well-being. Lastly, the construct of sensitivity and views on its structure need further substantive concretization.

Keywords Sensory processing sensitivity (SPS) · Psychological well-being · Ease of excitation · Low sensory threshold

1 Introduction

There are many points of view to the construct of sensitivity. Sensitivity is viewed as the readiness of an individual's affective reactions and subtle perception of the world around them (Batarshev, 2016). Some researchers view sensitivity as a personality feature of an individual which manifests itself in increased susceptibility to the events that happen to them and which is accompanied with increased anxiety, fear of new situations, people, and various kinds of challenges. Boterberg and Warreyn (2016) define sensitivity as a high sensitivity of the excitatory system and deep cognitive processing of physical, emotional, and social stimuli. Aron and Aron (1997), developing a Sensory processing sensitivity (SPS) theory, describe sensitivity as a temperamental feature that reflects how sensory information is transmitted to and processed by the brain. Sensitivity is proposed to be a genetic trait involving a deeper cognitive processing of stimuli that is driven by higher emotional reactivity. The authors claim that high sensitivity manifests in: (a) strong emotional reactivity (physiological stress reactivity, or arousability: it may be seen as an obstacle (Kernis, 2003) or an advantage (Baumeister et al., 2007) of deeper processing and general learning); (b) depth of cognitive processing (the highly sensitive individuals process internal and external stimuli more deeply than not sensitive people (Ahadi & Basharpoor, 2010; Jagiellowicz et al., 2010); (c) sensitivity to subtle detail (people with high levels of SPS are more observant of subtle features of their environment and as a result can be disturbed by high levels of stimulation, such as a loud noise, bright light, etc. (Aron, 2004); (d) susceptibility to excessive stimulation (it may manifest as a tendency to sensory overload and a desire to minimize a sensory stimulation (Benham, 2006; Evers et al., 2008).

Aron and Aron (1997) developed a special inventory—the Highly Sensitive Person Scale (HSPS) to measure sensitivity (Aron & Aron, 1997). In a series of studies, they found that SPS is a unidimensional construct (Aron & Aron, 1997). Hofmann and Bitran (2007), Neal et al. (2002) also confirmed the one-factor structure of SPS 'as the most parsimonious explanation of the data' (Neal et al., 2002, p. 367).

However, the other empirical findings do not support the assumption about the unidimensional factor structure of the HSPS. Evans and Rothbart (2008), Cheek et al. (2009) suggested a two-factor structure, Smolewska et al. (2006), Liss et al. (2008), Evers et al. (2008), Listou et al. (2016), and Konrad and Herzberg (2017) reported a three-factor solution. Other multi-factor solutions were originated from

Meyer et al. (2005) (four-factor structure), Blach and Egger (2014) (six-factor structure). The most common is the three-factor model of SPS, which includes 'ease of exitation', 'low sensory threshold', and 'aesthetic sensitivity' factors (Smolewska et al., 2006). Russian psychology has not yet developed an independent method for studying sensitivity, which is often included as a scale in personality or temperament questionnaires.

A series of studies showed that sensitivity is closely linked to negative psychological outcomes. Liss et al. (2008) identified that 'ease of excitation' and 'low sensory threshold' appear to represent the negative aspects of SPS because of their positive relations with anxiety and depression. Benham (2006) suggested the links between SPS and greater perceived stress, and more frequent symptoms of physical illness (such as bodily aches or pains to faintness and nausea). Hofmann and Bitran (2007) argued that sensory processing sensitivity is uniquely associated with the generalized subtype of social anxiety disorder, and the construct of SPS is highly correlated with harm avoidance and agoraphobic avoidance. SPS is also utilized to explain the high level of anxiety in certain individuals. For example, children with Autism-Spectrum Disorders are reported to have an elevated sensory sensitivity, coupled with the tendency to avoid physical sensation, that may lead to high levels of anxiety (Liss et al., 2008). Evers et al. (2008) proved that SPS is positively correlated with work stress, workload, emotional load, work displeasure, and need for recovery. In addition, SPS or its components are related to neurotic personality traits (Ahadi & Basharpoor, 2010; Smolewska et al., 2006). Russian psychologists studied sensitivity as a fear predisposition factor (Chernavsky, 2007), the internal determinant of marginal socialization of adolescents (Nikishina & Glushkova, 2009). At the same time, Aron et al. (2012) confirm that sensitive individuals manifest talent, good intuition, and high levels of integrity. Sensitivity is sometimes treated as a component of social creativity (Banyukhova & Shemelina, 2010). Smolewska et al. (2006) showed that individuals with high scores on Highly Sensitive Person Scale have deeper emotional response to positive reinforcement and have higher openness rate in the five-factor personality model.

It is known that personality plays a critical and influential role in predicting psychological well-being, satisfaction, adjustment, and quality of life (Anglim et al., 2020). Despite the fact that a variety of studies has been conducted in this field, there is no clear evidence of the role of sensitivity in psychological well-being that has been proposed as a series of psychological features involved in positive human functioning (Ryff, 1989). A literature review done by Abernethy (2010) maintains a hypothesis that sensory processing sensitivity may have a fundamental effect on the quality of life of highly sensitive individuals because of the coping mechanisms that they use to cope with these sensitivities. Evers et al. (2008) underlay the role of two subscale of SPS 'ease of excitation' and 'low sensory threshold' in the well-being decrease: they are negatively correlated with sense of coherence, comprehensibility, manageability, meaningfulness, and self-efficacy. On the other side, Sobocko and Zelenski (2015) point out that not all kinds of sensitivities lead to debilitating consequences: aesthetic (or orienting) sensitivity correlates more positively with psychological well-being.

Thus, a limited number of studies investigated the association of SPS with more desirable life outcomes.

In the present study we evaluated a Russian version of SPS scale with Aron and Aron scale as a starting point (Study 1) and assessed its associations with psychological well-being (Study 2).

2 Method

2.1 Participants and Procedure

Two approaches—active and passive—were employed to collect the field data: verbal advertising among undergraduate university students (i.e., 'snowball method'), and social media advertisements on Facebook and VK.com. Eventually 350 university students volunteers (233 females, 117 males between ages 17–25 years old, M age = 18.2, SD age = 1.7: M = 2,43 study year, SD = 1,04 contacted the laboratory of psychology in State University of Humanities and Social Studies and filled out the questionnaires. All participants received class extra credit for their participation. An additional group of 510 respondents (380 females and 130 males, aged 15–43, Mage = 22.6, SD age = 7.9 participated in anonymous online research (Google Forms). Thus a total of 860 respondents (613 females and 247 males aged 15–43, M age = 20,8, SD age = 3,56) filled out the questionnaires. The questionnaires were preceded by an informed consent form describing the research, data storage and processing conditions, and other ethical considerations. Only the data from participants who gave their informed consent was stored and used for further analysis.

2.2 Measures

2.2.1 Study 1

Highly Sensitive Person Scale (Aron & Aron, 1997) contains 27 statements each rated from 0 to 7 (0-'strongly disagree'; 7-'strongly agree') used to measure both physiological sensitivity to external factors (e.g., 'Loud noises create more discomfort to you than other people') and more subtle sensibility ('You are ill at ease when a lot happens simultaneously'). The questionnaire was translated into Russian by a professional translator and then edited by a team of psychologists (subject matter experts) with a command of English, so that the translated version fully matched the Russian cultural context. After that the proofread Russian version was translated back into English. The back translation and the original English version were cross-checked by a native English speaker (subject matter expert) to ensure that the original message of the questions was not lost in translation. The validity of the present questionnaire (Cronbach's alpha) was $\alpha = 0.83$ which is comparable to the results achieved in other studies $\alpha = 0.89$ (Smolewska et al., 2006); $\alpha = 0.85$ (Aron & Aron, 1997); $\alpha = 0.87$ (Hofmann & Bitran, 2007). Test–retest reliability was carried out as a part of validation procedure. Six months after the initial test 96 student volunteers took a sensitivity retest and the correlation coefficient for the test–retest was $r = 0.661$ at $p \leq 0.0001$.

2.2.2 Study 2

Psychological Well-Being Scale (RPWB) (Ryff, 1989, Russian version from Shevelenkova & Fesenko, 2005). The RPWB inventory consists of 84 questions rated from 0 to 6 (0-'totally disagree'; 6-'totally agree') reflecting the six areas of psychological well-being: 'Autonomy', 'Environmental mastery', 'Personal growth', 'Positive relations with others', 'Purpose in life', 'Self-acceptance'. The reliability of the Russian version of RPWB $\alpha = 0.59–0.81$ for scales that consist of 14 items (Shevelenkova & Fesenko, 2005), consistent with previous work in the present study $\alpha = 0.64–0.83$.

2.3 Analytical Plan

2.3.1. An exploratory and confirmatory analysis were conducted in Study 1 to develop the factor structure of Sensory Processing Sensitivity. The empirical samples was randomly split into two parts (430 cases in each group). An exploratory analysis (the hierarchical cluster analysis (ICLAST) (Revell 1979)) was conducted on a half of the sample than based on the results of the exploratory analysis a confirmatory factor analysis was conducted on the second half. The Lavaan 0.5–23.1097 software package was used for the model verification.

2.3.2. In Study 2 we divided all participants into 3 samples by the variable 'sensitivity' (M = 53, SD = 11,9): a sample with high sensitivity (N = 112), a sample with medium sensitivity (N = 630), and low sensitivity sample (N = 118). Subsequently, only the data of two contrast groups (low/high sensitivity) were used in the processing. To examine the effect of sensitivity on Psychological Well-being two-sample t-tests for independent samples were performed. Pearson correlation was used to examine the associations between sensitivity and psychological well-being. Statistical analyses were conducted in SPSS, 20.0.

Table 1 Fit Indices for the Two Factors and Three Factors Models

Model	χ^2	df, *p*	NNFI(TLI)	CFI	RMSEA	90%CI
2 K	86.93	61, 0.018	0.974	0.980	0.031	0.014–0.046
3K	293.83	132, 0.000	0.875	0.882	0.053	0.046–0.062

Note χ2. = chi-square statistics value, df = number of degrees of freedom, p = significance level, NNFI (TLI) = Non-normed Fit Index (Tucker-Lewis Index), CFI = Bentler Comparative Fit Index, RMSEA = Root Mean Square Error of Approximation, 90% CI = Confidence interval for RMSEA

3 Results

3.1 Study 1

The 'probing' clustering analysis allowed us to determine two sensitivity factors: C1 ($\alpha = 0.75$) and C2 ($\alpha = 0.81$), the selected clusters are very similar to the factors in Smolewska et al. (2006), Evans and Rothbart (2008), and Grimen and Diseth (2016) studies. The C1 cluster corresponds to the 'Low Sensory Threshold' subscale, and the C2 cluster corresponds to the—'Ease of Excitation' subscale.

Confirmatory factor analysis of the cross-validation sample (N = 430) was conducted to verify the bi or tri-factorial model with correlating factors. The models were evaluated using the WLSMV estimator (weighted least squares method), chi-square using Satorra-Bentler formula and robust evaluation of standard error. Model-data correlation values are given in Table 1.

The hierarchical cluster and confirmatory analyses employed for the operationalization procedure suggest that sensory processing sensitivity (SPS) can be described in a two-factors model consisting of 'Ease of Excitation' (EoE) and 'Low Sensory Threshold' (LST) subscales.

3.2 Study 2

Statistical analyses were conducted in SPSS, 20.0. The association between sensitivity and psychological well-being was tested with Pearson correlation, and t-tests were performed testing for differences in PWB scores for different levels of sensitivity. For these analyses, the variable 'Sensitivity' was divided into 3 samples (M = 53, SD = 11,9): a sample with high sensitivity (N = 112), a sample with medium sensitivity (N = 630), and low sensitivity sample (N = 118).

To examine the effect of sensitivity on Psychological well-being two-sample t-tests for independent samples (low/high sensitivity) were used (Table 2).

Table 2 Differences between low and high sensitive people on psychological well-being test

Psychological Well-Being	Low SPS		High SPS				
	M	SD	M	SD	df	t	p
Positive relations with others	62,42	13,80	57,77	9,81	212	2,93	0.00
Autonomy	61	13,76	53,34	9,73	211	4,85	0.00
Environmental mastery	60,47	14,04	55,95	8,48	194	2,94	0.00
Personal growth	61,93	13,60	65,11	5,69	159	−2,29	0.02
Purpose in life	63,14	15,35	64,21	8,08	179	−0,66	0.51
Self-acceptance	85,56	19,58	77,48	13,46	208	3,63	0.00
Psychological Well-Being	369,03	78,71	351,07	37,98	171	2,19	0.03

Note Low SPS = Low Sensory Processing Sensitivity sample, High SPS = High Sensory Processing Sensitivity sample

The significant differences in the level of psychological well-being in two samples were found: people with low sensitivity have a higher level of psychological well-being. There are no significant differences between the groups only in one scale 'purpose in life'.

The correlation analysis has shown that only one subscale of Psychological well-being ('personal growth') is disconnected with sensitivity (Table 3).

The 'ease of excitation' subscale of the HSPS is negatively correlated with five of the six subscales of the Psychological Well-being scale: 'positive relations with others' ($r = -0.292, p \leq 0.01$), 'autonomy' ($r = -0.330, p \leq 0.01$), 'environmental mastery' ($r = -0.182, p \leq 0.01$), 'purpose in life' ($r = -0.104, p \leq 0.01$), 'self-acceptance' ($r = -0.316, p \leq 0.01$). The 'low sensory threshold' subscale correlates with four parameters: 'positive relations with others' ($r = -0.165, p \leq$

Table 3 Correlations between highly sensitive person scale (HSPS) and psychological well-being (PWB)

Psychological well-being	HSPS	EoE	LST
Positive relations with others	−0.196**	−0.182**	−0.165**
Autonomy	−0.310**	−0.330**	−0.167**
Environmental mastery	−0.268**	−0.292**	−0.129**
Personal growth	−0.043	−0.038	−0.040
Purpose in life	−0.081*	−0.104**	−0.003
Self-acceptance	−0.280**	−0.316**	−0.112**

Note HSPS—Highly Sensitivity Person Scale (general index of SPS), EoE—'ease of excitation' subscale, LST—'low sensory threshold' subscale

**. Correlation is significant at the 0.01 level (2-tailed)

*. Correlation is significant at the 0.05 level (2-tailed)

0.01), 'autonomy' ($r = -0.167, p \leq 0.01$), 'environmental mastery' ($r = -0.129, p \leq 0.01$), 'self-acceptance' ($r = -0.112, p \leq 0.01$) of RPWB.

4 Discussion

This study aimed to operationalize the Russian version of HSPS and explore association between psychological well-being and sensory processing sensitivity.

Based on Study 1 the sensitivity was defined as a two-factors construct that manifests as an increased susceptibility to external and internal stimuli, which is expressed through negative emotional reactions and deep susceptibility (distress) to excessive stimulation (which is consistent with Evans and Rothbart (2008); Cheek et al. (2009). The results of this study did not confirm the one-dimensional model of sensitivity by Aron and Aron (1997), nor the three-factor model suggested by Smolevska et al. (2006). Current study of HSPS proved a two-factor model of sensitivity with 'ease of excitation' and 'low sensory threshold' subscales. Evans and Rothbart (2008) also viewed two highly correlated factors ('ease of excitation' and 'low sensory threshold'). The contents of these subscales are almost identical to the content of the similar subscales in Smolewska et al. (2006). Evans and Rothbart (2008) argued that the negative emotional response to sensory stimuli (the negative affectivity) have the most weight in the HSPS structure. The results of our study confirm their conclusions.

The third factor of HSPS, described by the other researchers (Smolewska et al., 2006; Liss et al., 2008; Evers et al., 2008; Konrad and Herzberg 2017) 'aesthetic sensitivity', which reflects the depth of cognitive processing of information and sensitivity to subtle detail identified in hierarchical cluster analysis showed week correlation with the other factors. Its content is irrelevant to the overall content of the HSPS questionnaire. Sobosko and Zelensky (2015) proved the distinct character of aesthetic sensitivity compared to other scales of SPS, in their study 'aesthetic sensitivity' showed the weakest correlations with the total HSPS and its other subscales. Thus, aesthetic sensitivity remains the most controversial factor in the structure of SPS, as evidenced by the fact that in many studies only the ease of excitation and the low sensory threshold subscales were correlated with self-efficacy manageability, meaningfulness, work stress, displeasure (Evers et al. 2008), anxiety, depression (Liss et al., 2005), poor social skills (Liss et al., 2008), avoidant personality disorder (Meyer & Carver, 2000), social phobia (Neal et al., 2002). The obtained results raise the question of revising the conceptual model of SPS developed by Aron and Aron (1997). Multiple studies have linked SPS with maladaptive outcomes: high level of anxiety and depression, low social skills, and avoidant personality disorder (Liss et al., 2005, Neal et al., 2002). The present study confirmed these findings. It was shown that high sensitivity may be seen as a factor of psychological well-being decrease.

The main features of the psychological well-being of highly sensitive people (HSP) are the following:

(a) difficulties in social contacts: it is hard for them to have warm, trusting relationships with others; they are usually isolated and disappointed, not ready to compromise in order to maintain the communication ('positive relations with others' scale of RPWB). The other studies (e.g., Aron & Aron, 1997, 2012; Liss et al., 2008) suggest that highly sensitive people often perceive their difficulties in contact with others as an internal limitation;
(b) low ability to resist social pressures, to think and act in particular ways, to regulate behavior from within, and evaluate themselves based on personal standards ('autonomy' scale of RPWB). Aron and Aron (1997) proposed that the strategy of dealing with environmental changes in SPS individuals connect with avoidant behavior caused by high autonomic arousal in response to new stimuli including social cue. As a result highly sensitive people often are seen as less logical and meaningful in their actions and self-efficacy (Aron & Aron, 1997; Evers et al., 2008;
(c) trouble in mastering everyday life, in controlling a complex array of external activities and advantage opportunities; in choosing or creating contexts, that suit needs and values ('environmental mastery' scale of RPWB).;
(d) a lot of criticism toward multiple aspects of themselves, including good and bad qualities and negative feelings about their past ('self-acceptance' scale of RPWB).
(e) at the same time, people with high sensitivity more than low sensitive people strive for development, realization of their potential, and improvement in themselves and behavior over time ('personal growth'). Aron and Aron (1997) theorized that some highly sensitive people seem to be able to take advantage of their sensitivities, some of them can be skilled cooks, visual artists, or musicians.

Obtained results correspond with the conclusions made by Listou Grimen et al. (2016), Meyer et al. (2005) toward the role of high sensitivity in a person's psychological health.

We found that both subscales of HSPS are closely negatively related to the psychological well-being of the individual, these results clarify and concretize the conclusions of Booth et al. (2015) who showed that high sensitivity may have a negative impact on the life satisfaction level. The present study suggests that the influence is manifested in a decrease of the psychological well-being level This conclusion is supported by Evans and Rothbart (2008), and Sobosko and Zelensky (2015) results demonstrating that high SPS lead to debilitating consequences. At the same time we point out the importance of further research of SPS construct and types of sensitivity, including aesthetic sensitivity, which, according to Aron and Aron (1997), and Sobosko and Zelensky (2015) can enhance a person's psychological well-being. Present findings provide potentially useful information for better understanding SPS and well-being.

5 Limitations

Because HSPS is a relatively new technique, there remain some aspects that need to be clarified and further studied. The empirical sample was relatively homogeneous in age and not sufficiently balanced by gender, the further research should continue on more heterogeneous groups. The absence of a randomized sample is another vulnerable part of the study. Nevertheless, in order to eliminate the errors associated with the lack of random selection of respondents, techniques of active and passive empirical sample formation were used.

The given assumption toward the association between the sensitivity and psychological well-being needs additional verification, including in the male and female samples. The present research was also limited by using only self-report measures. Future research might benefit by assessing sensitivity with physiological or behavioral measures. Future studies should expand research on SPS as a sensitivity marker to both positive and negative outcomes. Going beyond a correlational approach, more research is needed that manipulates the positive or negative impact of SPS on daily life, life satisfaction, and well-being in more controlled laboratory contexts or within intervention studies. Longitudinal study designs would allow a more in-depth analysis of causation and of differences at a within-person level, and the study of dynamic changes in SPS in connection to psychological well-being. Lastly, the construct of sensitivity and views on its structure need further substantive concretization.

References

Abernethy, H. (2010). The assessment and treatment of sensory defensiveness in adult mental health: A literature review. *British Journal of Occupational Therapy, 73*(5), 210–218. https://doi.org/10.4276/030802210X12734991664183

Ahadi, B., & Basharpoor, S. (2010). Relationship between sensory processing sensitivity, personality dimensions and mental health. *Journal of Applied Sciences, 10*, 570–574. https://doi.org/10.3923/jas.2010.570.574

Anglim, J., Horwood, S., Smillie, L. D., Marrero, R. J., & Wood, J. K. (2020). Predicting psychological and subjective well-being from personality: A meta-analysis. *Psychological Bulletin, 146*(4), 279. https://doi.org/10.1037/bul0000226

Aron, E. N. (2004). Revisiting Jung's concept of innate sensitiveness. *The Journal of Analytical Psychology, 49*, 337–367. https://doi.org/10.1111/j.1465-5922.2004.00465.x

Aron, E. N., & Aron, A. (1997). Sensory-processing sensitivity and its relation to introversion and emotionality. *Journal of Personality and Social Psychology, 73*, 345–368. https://doi.org/10.1037//0022-3514.73.2.345

Aron, E., Aron, A., & Jagiellowicz, J. (2012). Sensory processing sensitivity: A review in the light of the evolution of biological responsivity. *Personality and Social Psychology Review, 16*, 262–282. https://doi.org/10.1177/1088868311434213

Banyukhova, A. E., & Shemelina, O. S. (2010). Personality aspects of creativity. *Yaroslavl Pedagogical Bulletin, 2*(4), 205–211.

Batarshev, A. (2016). *Diagnosis of temperament and character.* St. Petersburg, Russia: Piter.

Baumeister, R. F., Vohs, K. D., Nathan DeWall, C., & Zhang, L. (2007). How emotion shapes behavior: Feedback, anticipation, and reflection, rather than direct causation. *Personality and Social Psychology Review, 11*(2), 167–203. https://doi.org/10.1177/1088868307301033

Benham, G. (2006). The highly sensitive person: Stress and physical symptom reports. *Personality and Individual Differences, 40*, 1433–1440. https://doi.org/10.1016/j.paid.2005.11.021

Booth, C., Standage, H., & Fox, E. (2015). Sensory-processing sensitivity moderates the association between childhood experiences and adult life satisfaction. *Personality and Individual Differences, 87*, 24–29. https://doi.org/10.1016/j.paid.2015.07.020

Boterberg, S., & Warreyn, P. (2016). Making sense of it all: The impact of sensory processing sensitivity on daily functioning of children. *Personality and Individual Differences, 92*, 80–86. https://doi.org/10.1016/j.paid.2015.12.022

Chernavsky, A. F. (2007). Psychophysiological preconditions for the manifestation of fear. *News of the Herzen's Russian State Pedagogical University, 19*(45), 11–19.

Evers, A., Rasche, J., & Schabracq, M. (2008). High sensory-processing sensitivity at work. *International Journal of Stress Management, 15*, 189–198. https://doi.org/10.1037/1072-5245.15.2.189

Hofmann, S. G., & Bitran, S. (2007). Sensory-processing sensitivity in social anxiety disorder: Relationship to harm avoidance and diagnostic subtypes. *Journal of Anxiety Disorders, 21*, 944–954. https://doi.org/10.1016/j.janxdis.2006.12.003

Jagiellowicz, J., Xu, X., Aron, A., Aron, E., Cao, G., Feng, T., & Weng, X. (2010). The trait of sensory processing sensitivity and neural responses to changes in visual scenes. *SCAN, 6*, 38–47. https://doi.org/10.1093/scan/nsq001

Kernis, M. H. (2003). Toward a conceptualization of optimal self-esteem. *Psychological Inquiry, 14*(1), 1–26. https://doi.org/10.1207/S15327965PLI1401_01

Liss, M., Mailloux, J., & Erchull, M. J. (2008). The relationship between sensory processing sensitivity, alexithymia, autism, depression, and anxiety. *Personality and Individual Differences, 45*, 255–259. https://doi.org/10.1016/j.paid.2008.04.009

Listou Grimen, H., & Diseth, Å. (2016). Sensory processing sensitivity: factors of the highly sensitive person scale and their relationships to personality and subjective health complaints. *Perceptual and Motor Skills, 123*(3), 637–653. https://doi.org/10.1177/0031512516666114

Meyer, B., Ajchenbrenner, M., & Bowles, D. P. (2005). Sensory sensitivity, attachment experiences, and rejection responses among adults with borderline and avoidant features. *Journal of Personality Disorders, 19*, 641–658. https://doi.org/10.1521/pedi.2005.19.6.641

Nikishina, V. B., & Glushkova, V. P. (2009). Internal determinants of the process of adolescents with ADHD socialization. *Izvestiya of Volgograd State Pedagogical University, 9*, 124–126.

Ryff, C. D. (1989). Happiness is everything, or is it? Explorations on the meaning of psychological well-being. *Journal of Personality and Social Psychology, 57*(6), 1069–1081.

Shevelenkova, T. D., & Fesenko, P. P. (2005). Psychological well-being (review of basic concepts and research methodology). *Psychological Diagnostics, 3*, 95–129.

Smolewska, K. A., McCabe, S. B., & Woody, E. Z. (2006). A psychometric evaluation of the highly sensitive person scale: The components of sensory-processing sensitivity and their relation to the BIS/BAS and "Big Five." *Personality and Individual Differences, 40*, 1269–1279. https://doi.org/10.1016/j.paid.2005.09.022

Sobocko, K., & Zelenski, J. M. (2015). Trait sensory-processing sensitivity and subjective well-being: Distinctive associations for different aspects of sensitivity. *Personality and Individual Differences, 83*, 44–49. https://doi.org/10.1016/j.paid.2015.03.045

Impact of a Digital Intervention Tool for Workplace Behavior and Emotional Wellbeing on Employees' Stress, Motivation, and Productivity

Himani Kulkarni, Christopher Chong, and Megan Lam

Abstract Digital interventions for mental health care are increasingly in demand as an accessible, personalized mental health tool. Their use in the workplace requires a deep dive into their efficacy and reliability. The study aims to study the efficacy and impact of bite-sized digital intervention tools on workplace stress, productivity, and motivation of employees. The study used a pretest–posttest randomized experimental design to assign employees ($n = 20$) to control or intervention groups. All participants answer the measures for workplace stress, productivity, and motivation at the beginning of the data collection. The control group responded to the measures again after a waiting time of seven days and the intervention group uses the digital intervention for seven days before responding to the same measures once more. The intervention group that used the digital intervention reported having significantly reduced stress, and increased motivation and productivity at the end of seven days in comparison to the control group. Further research with a variety of populations would be recommended. The present research can be utilized further to design digital interventions for other mental health outcomes.

Keywords Digital intervention · Employee stress · Employee motivation · Productivity

H. Kulkarni (✉) · M. Lam
Neurum Health, Hong Kong, China
e-mail: himani@neurumhealth.com
URL: https://www.neurumhealth.com

M. Lam
e-mail: meg@neurumhealth.com
URL: https://www.neurumhealth.com

H. Kulkarni · C. Chong
University of Birmingham, Birmingham, UK
e-mail: cxc1117@student.bham.ac.uk

P. Macaulay and L. Tan (eds.), *Applied Psychology Readings*,
https://doi.org/10.1007/978-981-99-2613-8_6

1 Introduction

Workplace stress and reduced productivity are a concern for both employers and employees. Lowered motivation and employee engagement cause emotional and financial distress to the employees and the workplace. Employees struggle to meet their professional goals and employers suffer financial and credibility loss. The material cost for productivity loss due to employee absenteeism can reach up to an annual cost of HK$550 million to HK$860 million. More broadly, the total annual financial cost of workplace stress was concluded to be HK$4.81 billion to HK$7.09 billion (Siu et al., 2020 Nov 19). The economic cost is a significant marker of the need for workplace interventions aimed at reducing such losses for employees and employers both. Employees report concerns related to workload, interpersonal conflicts, constraints at the workplace, and worries around job insecurity as significant factors that lead to productivity loss and absenteeism at the workplace (Van Der Feltz-Cornelis et al., 2020). These outcomes also increase the load of medical expenses for the employee as well as the organization. A report by McKinsey & Company (July 8, 2021) states that 75 out of 100 employees require support to strengthen and foster their mental health. Another 24 would have a moderate need for psychotherapy and 1 of every 100 would need more acute mental health intervention. This loss of productivity especially when the employees are present in the workplace is attributed to physical and mental health challenges apart from the workplace concerns like workload and interpersonal conflict (Brassey et al., 2021).

The workplace wellness programs that were once considered a luxury and a favor, have now been recognized as a necessity and a consequential factor of investment plans. The organizations are deliberate in understanding the scope of such programs in reducing economic costs, improving employee performance and motivation, and retaining talent. This shift in the understanding of workplace stress, and motivation, has been found to impact productivity positively. Organizations have been employing a variety of interventions to contribute to healthier and more competent workplaces (Howarth et al., 2018 May 10). More recently, the interventions are also digitally implemented and attempt to bridge the gap between the employee and the resource. Several mobile applications and websites have attempted to create programs that can be delivered to the end user with lesser barriers while maintaining integrity and credibility. This can form a vital step in the direction of private, accessible, and affordable mental health care for the end user.

In an ever-developing society, web-based programs and interventions that aim to benefit the user's mental health have become increasingly popular over the past decade. Several extremely promising studies have helped support the success as well as the efficacy of such programs in reducing emotional distress and improving psychological health (Inkster, 2018; Lappalainen, 2013). While most studies focus on mental health and clinical concerns such as depression, anxiety, and stress, there is growing evidence in support of using digital interventions for workplace concerns such as decreased motivation, perceived workload, digital and office workspaces, and interpersonal conflict at work. The digital interventions range from meditation and positive affirmation to cognitive restructuring and empathetic chatbots.

Digital interventions attempt to make mental health intervention more accessible, affordable, and free of social barriers that exist in accessing mental health care. The digital interventions are set to fill in the shoes of traditional mental health care such as therapists and coaches, as well as psychiatrists and clinical psychologists. This brings up the question of how the interventions can form a space akin to therapeutic alliance and rapport that the human connection forms. Digital interventions have been attempting to fulfill this need for accessible mental health resources with the help of artificial intelligence and guiding tools.

The present study aims to understand the impact of an app-based self-paced digital intervention on workplace stress, productivity, and motivation in an attempt to address the gap that was noticed in the available research. Recognizing the reach, accessibility, and cost-effective nature of such interventions, this study aims to understand their efficacy on the aforementioned behavioral health indicators.

2 Methodology

2.1 Design

The design of the study is a quasi-experimental design aimed at understanding the impact of the digital intervention between the intervention and the control group and the pre- and post-assessment. The intervention group used the digital intervention tools for seven days between the pre- and post-assessments, while the control group did not engage in any intervention in the period between pre- and post-assessments.

2.2 Sample

The study has a sample of $N = 20$ participants which are equally split between control and intervention groups. The sample was collected through convenience sampling and purposive snowballing techniques. The sample was split randomly into two equal groups for intervention and control where $N = 10$ each. The participants are employed full-time and have been in the workplace for six months or more. The participants are between 20 and 40 years of age and are not matched for gender. The employees who are retiring in the next year are also excluded. All participants belong to the working population of Hong Kong.

2.3 Intervention

The intervention is a digital intervention tool on the Neurum app designed to impact stress, productivity, and motivation at the workplace. The tools are a digital module consisting of smaller sessions that each focus on a different concern and kind of therapeutic model. The intervention focuses on six core areas: (a) negative cognition, (b) self-blame, (c) social support, (d) bodily reaction to stress, (e) healthy coping strategies, and (f) recognition of the problem.

Negative cognition is defined as the thinking patterns that lead to stress and unhealthy practices. *Self-blame* is understood as the tendency to blame the self for problems and failure at the workplace. *Social support* is described as the perceived support available to help with stressful situations. *Bodily reactions* to stress are the natural response to stress that can be observed physically and measured objectively. *Healthy coping strategies* are practices and perspectives that help in dealing with stressful situations and are helpful in the long run. *Recognition of the problem* is the ability to notice discomfort and understand the reasons for it.

The tools derive techniques from five different schools of therapy. The techniques are (A) psychoeducation, (B) Somatic techniques, (C) Cognitive techniques, (D) Person-Centered techniques, and (E) Positive Psychology Techniques.

The bite-sized nature of the sessions aims to make the tools accessible for the users by reducing the effort and time it takes to reach personalized mental health guidance suited for ecological environments.

2.4 Research Tools

The tools are three scales used to measure the scores for workplace stress, productivity, and motivation at the workplace. The scale used for workplace stress is the 21-question Work Stress Questionnaire (WSQ) (Frantz & Holmgren, 2019 Nov 27), 18 Questions from the Individual Work Performance Questionnaire for productivity at the workplace (Ramos-Villagrasa et al., 2019), and 12 questions from The Motivation at Work Scale (MAWS) (Gagné et al., 2010).

2.5 Data Analysis Tool

The data is analyzed using a paired *t*-test to look for any significant differences between the scores of the participants in the intervention and control group and pre- and post-assessment.

3 Results

The data collected from the four groups (intervention and control, pre- and post-assessments) was analyzed using descriptive statistics and the *t*-test was employed to understand the statistical difference and to check whether there is a statistically significant difference between the scores obtained for the intervention group after the intervention was delivered. The scores obtained and compared for the four groups are presented in the tables below (see Table 1).

The table shows the mean scores, standard deviation, standard error of the mean, and 95% confidence interval lower and upper limits for the three measures of the intervention group, both pre- and post-assessment. The mean scores for the three measures are 2.00 for work stress, 2.80 for productivity at work, and 2.0 for motivation at work. The standard deviation for stress at work is 1.76, for productivity at the workplace is 4.61, and that for motivation at work is 2.9 in this group (see Table 2).

The table shows the *t*-score, degree of freedom, and *p*-value for the intervention group, pre- and post-assessment. The *p*-values for stress at work for the pre- and post-assessment are 0.03, that for productivity at the workplace is 0.044, and that for workplace motivation is 0.031. All three values show valid change as they are $P < 0.05$. The *p*-values indicate that there is a significant change between the scores obtained for stress, productivity, and motivation between the pre- and post-assessment for the intervention group (see Table 3).

Table 1 Paired samples test of the intervention group showing mean, standard deviation, standard error of mean, and confidence interval ($N = 10$)

		Mean	Std. deviation	Std. error mean	95% confidence interval lower	95% confidence interval upper
Pair 1	StressPre–StressPost	2.00000	1.76383	0.55777	0.73823	3.26177
Pair 2	ProductivityPre–ProductivityPost	2.80000	4.61399	1.45907	0.50065	6.10065
Pair 3	MotivationPre–MotivationPost	2.00000	2.98142	0.94281	0.13278	4.13278

Table 2 Paired samples test of the intervention group showing *t* score, degree of freedom, and *p*-value of significance ($N = 10$)

		t	df	One-sided p
Pair 1	StressPre–StressPost	3.586	9	0.003
Pair 2	ProductivityPre–ProductivityPost	1.919	9	0.044
Pair 3	MotivationPre–MotivationPost	2.121	9	0.031

Table 3 Paired samples test of the control group showing mean, standard deviation, standard error of mean, and confidence interval ($N = 10$)

		Mean	Std. deviation	Std. error mean	95% confidence interval lower	95% confidence interval upper
Pair 1	StressPre–StressPost	0.20000	6.44291	2.03743	−4.40898	4.80898
Pair 2	ProductivityPre–ProductivityPost	4.60000	7.12117	2.25191	−9.69418	0.49418
Pair 3	MotivationPre–MotivationPost	5.00000	10.13246	3.20416	−12.24832	2.24832

Table 4 Paired samples test of the control group showing t score, degree of freedom, and p-value of significance ($N = 10$)

		t	df	One-sided p
Pair 1	StressPre–StressPost	0.098	9	0.462
Pair 2	ProductivityPre–ProductivityPost	−2.043	9	0.036
Pair 3	MotivationPre–MotivationPost	−1.560	9	0.077

The table shows the mean scores, standard deviation, standard error of the mean, and 95% confidence interval lower and upper limits for the three measures of the control group, both pre- and post-assessment. The mean scores for the three measures are 0.20 for work stress, −4.60 for productivity at work, and −5.00 for motivation at work. The standard deviation for stress at work is 6.44, for productivity at the workplace is 7.12, and that for motivation at work is 10.13 in this group (see Table 4).

The table shows the t-score, degree of freedom, and p-value for the control group, pre- and post-assessment. The p-values for stress at work for the pre- and post-assessment are 0.46, that for productivity at the workplace is 0.036, and that for workplace motivation is 0.07. Two of the values (workplace stress and motivation) show no observable change as they are $P > 0.05$. The p-values indicate that there is no significant change between the scores obtained for stress, and motivation between the pre- and post-assessment for the intervention group.

4 Discussion

The study aimed to understand the impact of the digital intervention tools on the Neurum app on work-related stress, productivity, and motivation at the workplace. The result obtained indicates that the p-value for the intervention group is statistically significant at a 95% confidence interval. The p-values for stress at work for the score pre- and post-assessment is 0.03, that for productivity at the workplace is 0.044, and that for workplace motivation is 0.031. All three values show an observable change in the scores obtained on the measures of workplace stress, productivity, and motivation after the intervention is delivered in the form of self-paced digital tools over seven days. It can be safely argued that employing digital intervention contributed to reduced stress, increased motivation, and productivity at the workplace.

The stress at the workplace reduces after the use of the digital intervention for the given sample. The stress likely decreased due to a variety of factors both internal and external. The design of the tools could have contributed to reducing stress in a few different ways. The tools are created in a friendly and supportive language that is easy to comprehend and follow. The self-paced design of the tools would likely be easy to schedule on a busy day. The guided practices likely provide direction and support to try out a new behavior, thinking patterns, and social relationships. Digital intervention tools that show flexibility and convenience for both the interventionists and the recipient have been seen to be more effective in impacting behavior and behavioral health (Marcu et al., 2022 Mar 30).

Productivity and motivation increase post the use of the digital intervention hinting at the impact of the intervention delivered among other external factors. The tools likely have impacted negative thinking patterns and reduced internal barriers that inhibited productivity and motivation. A significant argument for presenteeism or the loss of productivity when the employee is present is the conflict in interpersonal relationships people have at the workplace, whether it is with their managers or colleagues (Van Der Feltz-Cornelis et al., 2020). The intervention dealt with social support and self-esteem at the workplace, guiding people through gaining better insight and altering behavior to resolve conflicts and improve the quality of their time at the workplace. Research shows that digital interventions that are easy to comprehend and have measures for accessibility are much more likely to be effective in imparting emotional and behavioral changes (Marcu et al., 2022 Mar 30).

Digital interventions are most useful when they are creative and cognizant of the changes, they can bring about in health care (Michie et al., 2017 Jun 29). It is likely that the interventions effectively impacted the measures in this study because of the nature of the delivery. Modules that can be accessed on people's own devices with little regulation or monitoring from those around them are likely to feel private, and safe, and bypass the stigma that comes with asking for emotional help (Marcu et al., 2022 Mar 30). This can pave way for higher adherence to the intervention plan and increased sense of privacy and safety for the user.

The impact on one of the measures would likely have positively impacted the other two, given the observed relationship between stress, motivation, and productivity at the workplace. Reduced stress is likely to be a factor in increasing motivation and productivity at the workplace (Bui et al., 2021 Feb 12). Similarly, increased motivation is likely to reduce stress and increase productivity in the workplace (Shkoler & Kimura, 2020).

The control group shows an increase in productivity but no significant change in motivation or stress levels. It is likely that the group became more cognizant of their productivity levels or defined it differently in different sectors leading to these results in the control group.

5 Limitations and Implication

The study can help evaluate and understand the creation of similar digital interventions combating issues both in and out of the workplace. The study would need to be replicated with a larger and more diverse population, to examine the efficacy of the said interventions. This study could inspire further studies to investigate the reliability and efficacy of the digital intervention programs available across platforms in different areas of emotional distress. The present research paves way for future research on not just the reduction of emotional distress, but for outcomes related to the quality of life and fulfilment in various contexts.

6 Conclusion

The purpose of the study was to understand the impact of the digital intervention on the Neurum app on the stress, productivity, and motivation of the employees at the workplace. The design of the study was a quasi-experiment design employed to study the differences between the control and intervention groups and the pre- and post-assessments. The digital intervention was a self-paced app-based intervention focusing on varied components of workplace behavior and experience. The tools used to measure the change were three standardized scales used to measure workplace stress (Work Stress Questionnaire—WSQ), productivity (Individual Work Performance Questionnaire), and motivation (The Motivation at Work Scale—MAWS). The change observed for the intervention group was statistically significant from the other groups. The impact observed could be attributed to the design, content, and accessibility of the tools among other external factors. The change observed for the control group was not statistically significant for any measure except productivity.

References

Brassey, J., Güntner, A., Issak, K., & Silberzahn, T. (2021). *Using digital tech to support employees' mental health and resilience.* McKinsey & Company.

Bui, T., Zackula, R., Dugan, K., & Ablah, E. (2021). Workplace stress and productivity: A cross-sectional study. *Kansas Journal of Medicine, 14*, 42–45. https://doi.org/10.17161/kjm.vol141 3424. PMID: 33654542; PMCID: PMC7889069.

Frantz, A., & Holmgren, K. (2019). The work stress questionnaire (WSQ)-reliability and face validity among male workers. *BMC Public Health, 19*(1):1580. https://doi.org/10.1186/s12889-019-7940-5. PMID: 31775694; PMCID: PMC6882173.

Gagné, M., Forest, J., Gilbert, M. H., Aubé, C., Morin, E., & Malorni, A. (2010). The motivation at work scale: Validation evidence in two languages. *Educational and Psychological Measurement*, *70*, 628–646. https://doi.org/10.1177/0013164409355698

Howarth, A., Quesada, J., Silva, J., Stephanie, J. (2018). The impact of digital health interventions on health-related outcomes in the workplace: A systematic review. *Digit Health, 4*, 2055207618770861. https://doi.org/10.1177/2055207618770861. PMID: 29942631; PMCID: PMC6016571.

Inkster, B. S. (2018). An empathy-driven, conversational artificial intelligence agent (Wysa) for digital mental well-being: Real-world data evaluation mixed-methods study. *JMIR mHealth and uHealth, 6*(11), e12106.

Lappalainen, P. K. (2013). Feasibility of a personal health technology-based psychological intervention for men with stress and mood problems: Randomized controlled pilot trial. *JMIR Research Protocols, 2*(1), e1. https://doi.org/10.2196/resprot.2389

Marcu, G., Ondersma, S., Spiller, A., Broderick, B., Kadri, R., & Buis, L. (2022). The perceived benefits of digital interventions for behavioral health: Qualitative interview study. *Journal of Medical Internet Research, 24*(3), e34300. https://doi.org/10.2196/34300. PMID: 35353045; PMCID: PMC9008533.

Michie, S., Yardley, L., West, R., Patrick, K., & Greaves, F. (2017). Developing and evaluating digital interventions to promote behavior change in health and health care: Recommendations resulting from an international workshop. Journal of *Medical Internet Research, 19*(6), e232. https://doi.org/10.2196/jmir.7126. PMID: 28663162; PMCID: PMC5.

Ramos-Villagrasa, P. J., Barrada, J., Fernández-del-Río, E., & Koopmans, L. (2019). Assessing job performance using brief self-report scales: The case of the individual work performance questionnaire. *Journal of Work and Organizational Psychology, 35*, 195–205. https://doi.org/10.5093/jwop2019a21

Shkoler, O., & Kimura, T. (2020). How does work motivation impact employees' investment at work and their job engagement? A moderated-moderation perspective through an international lens. *Frontiers in Psychology*. https://doi.org/10.3389/fpsyg.2020.00038

Siu, O. L., et al. (2020). Occupational stress and its economic cost in Hong Kong: The role of positive emotions. *International Journal of Environmental Research and Public Health, 17*(22), 8601.

Van Der Feltz-Cornelis, C., Varley, D., Allgar, V., & de Beurs, E. (2020). Workplace stress, presenteeism, absenteeism, and resilience amongst university staff and students in the COVID-19 lockdown. *Frontiers in Psychiatry, 11*, 588803. https://doi.org/10.3389/fpsyt.2020.588803

Men in Dating: Exploring Indonesian Men's Experience in Dating Relationships

Karel Karsten Himawan and Pradipta Christy Pratiwi

Abstract Current body of literature has consistently suggested that men's voice in research around romantic relationships is underrepresented. The cultural representation around gender in society, particularly those in a patriarchal culture that seems to polarize men against the relationship being, also adds to the hesitancy of men in having their voices heard in discourses about relationships and romance. On the other side, growing evidence indicates how men construct, perceive, and experience romantic relationships in a unique way compared to women. The present study aims at exploring men's unique perception and experience, particularly in a dating relationship. Seven heterosexual males participated in a 120-min, onsite focus group discussion. Participants' responses were audio recorded and their responses were transcribed for analysis through thematic coding procedure. Three themes are identified highlighting men's perceptions and experience in a relationship: (1) relationship as a means for self-validation and self-existence, (2) relationship as a long-term journey, and (3) common societal misconceptions of men's roles in a relationship. The results challenged common stereotypes among men and the traditional hypergamy marriage ideal. The study adds important contribution in providing nuances in men's experience in a relationship beyond the discussion of power and sex, which were often the predominant themes as indicated in previous literature. Practically termed, the study provides valuable insights to improve well-being of individuals of both genders by managing and aligning their relationship expectations.

K. K. Himawan (✉)
Faculty of Psychology, Universitas Pelita Harapan, Tangerang, Indonesia
e-mail: karel.karsten@uph.edu
URL: https://www.uph.edu

RELASI Research Lab, Universitas Pelita Harapan, Tangerang, Indonesia

Faculty of Medicine, The University of Queensland, Brisbane, Australia

P. C. Pratiwi
Department of Psychology, Universitas Negeri Semarang, Semarang City, Indonesia
e-mail: pradiptacp@mail.unnes.ac.id
URL: https://www.unnes.ac.id

P. Macaulay and L. Tan (eds.), *Applied Psychology Readings*,
https://doi.org/10.1007/978-981-99-2613-8_7

Keywords Dating · Marriage · Masculinity · Patriarchal · Relationship · Romantic

1 Introduction

Happy wife, happy life.

Such a popular quote believed by current society picks our attention. While some people believe that this quote captures quite accurately how a man really defines well-being in their relationship, this begs a question: *is a man's well-being in a romantic relationship solely, or heavily, dependent on their partner?*

It is not surprising to have an impression that emotional nuances in the romantic relationship seem to be more dominated from women's perspective. Current literature supports this notion by highlighting the feminist view in defining the experience of dating (Smith-Hefner, 2005), partnership (Vignato, 2012), marriage (Huang, 2017), or relationship abstinence (Simpson, 2015). Minimal research has been conducted to explore such an experience from masculinity perspective. A scoping review was conducted to explore how current body of knowledge draw an experience of romantic relationship from masculinity perspective in the last ten years (Himawan et al., 2022b). A total of 164 studies were extracted. The result confirms our presumption that power and sex are the two dominant themes that explain how romantic relationship is experienced through masculinity perspective. Men tend to misuse their dominant role by acting as perpetrators of violence in their romantic relationships, especially related to sexual harassment. In other words, man is pictured as an oversexed, emotionally restraint, creature (Healey, 2020).

The consistent picture of man as captured by current literature may indicate two things. On one side, it depicts the accurate nature of man as a less emotional being with higher sexual arousal than woman. On the other side, there is a possibility that some research is reframed around the strong patriarchal gender stereotype that is embedded in the society. In other words, we cannot be sure to what extent the male representation in the current literature is affected by the entrenched gender stereotype. This is particularly challenging given that women tend to be more responsive in study participation (Kalmijn & Liefbroer, 2010; Slauson-Blevins & Johnson, 2016), which makes men's voices even less heard. Furthermore, some research seems to take various problems associated with the abuse of power in sexual activities as its point of departure (Fekih-Romdhane et al., 2022; Henao et al., 2022; Langton et al., 2017). Interpersonal and sexual violence, where man is positioned as the perpetrator, accounts for more than a quarter of the available literature that describes a man's experience in romance (Himawan et al., 2022b). While this might represent the consistently high prevalence of interpersonal violence (Sardinha et al., 2022), focusing only on the problematic side of the experience might give a short-sighted view about what a man perceives, and how a man experiences a romantic relationship. Therefore, a neutral perspective is needed to explore the experience of a romantic relationship from a man's perspective (Himawan, 2022; Himawan et al., 2022b). We incorporate this attitude in our current study by letting men defines the "experience" rather than constructing the experience from the problems observed in the society, which is very deeply rooted in strong patriarchal gender stereotype.

While there is much to explore about how men experience, perceive, and expect from a romantic relationship, the current study aims to articulate men's voices in the experience and expectation of a romantic relationship. Considering the strong cultural influence in the social representation of gender, we choose dating relationship as the context for this preliminary study.

Indonesia provides an interesting window to explore how masculinity is negotiated in dating relationship. In Indonesia, dating (*pacaran*) is considered a significant step toward marriage (Himawan et al., 2021a), and hence a temporary status. Casual dating is rarely acknowledged in Indonesia, as society upholds the normativity of marriage (Himawan et al., 2018b), with no social favorability attached to marriage alternatives, such as cohabitation (Hull, 2016). Long-term courtship is seen as being vulnerable to sexual promiscuity (*zina*) (Bennett, 2005; Himawan et al., 2021a). Taken as a committed form of relationship, an individual needs to formally propose to their partner before commencing into their dating relationship (Himawan et al., 2021a). We believe the unique cultural representation attached to dating relationship would reveal an interesting perspective regarding how Indonesian men experience their relationship.

Gender Stereotypes in Dating Relationship: The Indonesian Perspective

Cultural practices about dating relationship in Indonesia is less studied, hence literature is limited to capture such a dynamic, particularly from a masculinity perspective. However, from the available literature, two patterns emerged related to gender expectations in dating relationship.

First, many Indonesian people favor the hypergamy ideal of marriage, and this implies dating practices. Marriage according to hypergamy ideal occurs between a male partner with higher socioeconomic status and a female with lower status than that of male (Utomo, 2012). This form of marriage acknowledges male superiority. While many Indonesian women nowadays challenge the male superiority and demand gender equality in various social contexts, such as participation in work and education (Himawan et al., 2019). Interestingly many women still favorably perceive male superiority in marital relationships. Such a persisting favorable attitude toward hypergamy ideal may be socially and religiously conditioned as Indonesian Marriage Law as well as Islamic and Christianity teachings, the two major religions in Indonesia, position husband as the family leader and provider (Himawan et al., 2018a; Utomo, 2012). In dating practices, upholding to hypergamy ideal means that man should be the one who initiates (propose) the relationship to woman (in Indonesia this is called "*menembak*") (Himawan et al., 2021a). Nevertheless, such a perception tends to be articulated from women's perspective. This notion is supported by studies highlighting how some unmarried women felt that they lost in the market because no man was approaching her, or that they intentionally concealed their career position or their higher education degree so that a man will not be threatened to approach her

(Himawan, 2020). To our knowledge, no literature has revealed the man's attitude about this perception.

Secondly, Indonesian men are presumed to only expect short-time fulfillment in their dating relationship, while women are aiming toward a long-term commitment. This claim is supported by worldwide literature (He & Tsang, 2017; McKeown, 2015), but is also evident in Indonesia (Vignato, 2012). Belief that men only look for short-term fulfillment (i.e. sexual satisfaction) motivates some women to be highly careful in the mate selection (Vignato, 2012), and expect courtship to be shortly followed by marriage. The short temporality of courtship is significant for women, especially in Indonesia, given the narrow age range where a woman is considered normative single (between 20 and 30 years) (Himawan et al., 2021a; Jones, 2010). Hence, courtship is considered risky for some women because, if their relationship breaks up after they pass the normative single period, they will be at risk of stigma due to being single and overcome significant challenges to encounter a new partner (Himawan et al., 2021a). Again, this assumption was constructed from the women's assumption of man (Himawan, 2020; Vignato, 2012) and no studies have highlighted the Indonesian men's view of dating relationship.

Study Focus

Given the limited available literature that explores experience in dating relationship from men's perspective, the current study aims to reveal Indonesian man's view, experience, and expectation about dating relationship. This exploratory study is set as a preliminary study utilizing a small number of individuals through focus group discussion to facilitate a neutral, genuine exploration. The research question of this study is: *How do men experience, perceive, and expect from their dating relationship?*

2 Methods

Design. We conducted semi-structured focus group discussion to explore the perceptions and experiences of Indonesian men in dating relationships. Focus group discussion is used in qualitative research to obtain various information or to describe an experience based on individual perceptions (Sandelowski, 2000). In particular, focus group method is considered appropriate as it incorporates the three characteristics highlighting the merits of focus group discussion (Powell & Single, 1996): little is known about the topic (manhood perspective in dating experience especially from patriarchal culture), the topic needs to be explored from different points of view (religion, sociocultural background, educational background might be involved in men's conceptualization of romantic relationship), complex variables were involved and needs to be reduced to the most essential ones (the key themes accounting for men's experience and expectation in dating) Indonesia. The interaction among participants enabled through focus group discussions encourages them to build rich reflection on the aspects of life being studied (Acocella, 2012).

Participants and recruitment. We recruited participants using purposive sampling, with the following criteria: (1) having a minimum age of 27 years (27 years are often used as a cutoff age where marriage becomes normative in Indonesia Himawan et al., 2021a, 2021b), (2) were in a heterosexual dating relationship at the time of participating, and (3) lived in Jakarta and surrounding areas.

Seven participants responded to our advertisement and attended the focus group discussion. The number is considered ideal for research using focus group discussions (Bloor et al., 2000; Wilkerson et al., 2014). The age range of participants in this focus group discussion ranged from 27 to 32 years, a typical age range for Indonesian participants to be in the "dating" milestone prior to marriage (Jones, 2018). Participants had a minimum of high school educational background, while most of them ($n = 5$) were university graduates. Six participants were employees in private and public sectors, and the remaining one was an entrepreneur. Table 1 presents summary of participants' characteristics.

From the time of recruitment for 2 weeks, we disseminated information about this research using flyers. The flyer contains an invitation to join in the discussion about men's perceptions of relationships. We also take advantage of Facebook advertising and post flyers on social media to reach a wider audience of participants.

We obtained seven participants to be involved in the focus group discussion. Before starting the focus group discussion, participants were asked to fill out and sign an informed consent, as an agreement to participate in this study.

Materials. The list of questions used in the focus group discussion was discussed by all authors. Questions were formulated based on the insights of the previously conducted scoping review. There were three focuses of the discussion: dating conceptualisation, dating experience, and dating expectation. In dating conceptualisation, participants were asked to share their perception of romantic relationship (*What is a romantic relationship for you? How important is romantic relationship for you?*). In dating experience, participants were asked to share their pleasant and unpleasant dating experience (*Please share your pleasant experience in dating*). In the last section of dating expectation, participants were asked to share what they consider an ideal type of partner (*What is an ideal image of a romantic partner to you?*). In this section, participants were also asked about any social misperception that they

Table 1 Participant demographics and characteristics

Participant ID	Age	Highest education	Occupation	Religion	Ethnicity
C-01	32	Senior high school	Teacher	Islam	Javanese
C-02	27	Senior high school	Entrepreneur	Islam	Javanese
C-03	28	Bachelor degree	Employee	Islam	Sundanese
C-04	29	Bachelor degree	Employee	Islam	Javanese
C-05	29	Bachelor degree	Employee	Christian	Chinese
C-06	27	Bachelor degree	Civil servant	Not answered	Betawi
C-07	28	Diploma degree	Employee	Islam	Padang

perceived about men in romance (*Is there any social misperception about men that you believe to be inaccurate? Would you share?*).

The question format was adapted to the recommended format for qualitative research: each question is designed to trigger a series of related specific questions or issues (Corbin & Strauss, 2015). A set of questions that were prepared focuses on two areas: participants' experience in dating and participants' expectation in dating. Given its exploratory nature, we maintained a naturalistic inquiry to allow participants to reveal the themes based on their actual experience.

Procedure. Study advertisement was conducted utilizing Facebook and Instagram paid advertisement. Advertisement was tailored to only appear to users that corresponded to the study criteria. Advertisement was conducted two weeks prior to the actual date of discussion. In the study advertisement, interested individuals were asked to indicate their interest by completing a short online survey.

The online survey has two parts. The first part contained study information, nature of participation, risks and mitigation, and ethical clearance of the study. If individuals agreed with the information, they were asked to provide a digital consent by clicking the agree button. Digital agreement was required before they were able to access the second part of the survey. The second part collected participants' demographic characteristics, including age, educational background, occupation, and dating duration. They were also asked to indicate their email address or phone number to be further contacted should their responses match the study criteria. Nine eligible participants were invited and seven of them confirmed their attendance.

The discussion was conducted in Indonesian language, in a hotel located in the central Jakarta for practical access for participants. A moderator was assigned based on the gender similarity to the studied group, which was the first author of this paper. The moderator has completed training in qualitative research and has extensive experience in conducting qualitative studies. The discussion was audio and video recorded and lasted for 121 min. We asked participants' consent for video recording to enable non-verbal observation in the data analysis. All participants provided consent. Given the sensitive nature of the topic, no other researcher team member was present in the discussion, except a moderator and seven participants. Seating arrangement was designed in a U-shape, with moderator sitting in the center. Participants were rewarded a cash amount of IDR 250.000, for participating to cover their transportation cost and to appreciate their time and thoughts.

Data Analysis. Recordings were professionally transcribed verbatim before being analyzed. The second author watched the video recording and took note of the important points for analysis.

Qualitative thematic analysis guided the analysis process. We performed dynamic form of analysis of both verbal and visual data, to enable comprehensive and rich interpretation. Both authors first read the transcripts to get a picture of the participants' experience. We examined the meaning units in the transcript and eliminated redundant meaning units. The meaning unit was then transformed into psychological meaning (Sandelowski, 2000). Results were organized into themes based on the scope of the issues. Participants' identity was masked and coded to maintain confidentiality. Selected verbatims that were used to articulate the themes were translated by the authors.

Ethics

This ethical component of this research was approved by *Konsorsium Psikologi Ilmiah Nusantara* (KPIN) with ethical clearance number 065/2022.

3 Results

All participants equally participated in the discussion. Many participants approached the moderator before the discussion commenced, reflecting that they highly welcomed the research as they felt that many studies around this topic tended to only focus on women.

Participants did not know each other before the discussion. The moderator started the discussion by asking each participant to briefly introduce himself by mentioning their name and occupation. After a brief introduction, the moderator asked participants to describe their perception of romantic relationship. No rigid order was expected for participants to share their thoughts. The advantage of utilizing focus group discussion was articulated by a participant who indicated that

> I initially did not want to bring about this issue because I thought that might be just me [who think that way].. But then after you talked, I feel that I am alone and I really want to speak this up.

The participant mentioned about his presumed unpopular belief that in his relationship, he tried not to play a dominating role. In that sense, he wanted to give up the "*authority as a man to decide*" and to value partner participation in decision making.

Three themes emerged reflecting the participants' experience of dating relationship from Indonesian perspective: relationship as a means for self-validation and self-existence, relationship as a long-term journey, and common societal misconceptions of men's roles in a relationship. To keep the paper succinct, original verbatim was excluded from the report, and only English-translated verbatim was provided.

Theme 1: Relationship as a means for self-validation and self-existence. All participants appeared to value their romantic relationships as important for their self-validation and self-existence. Dating relationships helped participants to better understand themselves, in particular their values and identity. This is particularly reflected when a moderator asked: "*what was missing should you were not in a relationship right now?*" Participants C-02 answered,

> my existence.. I would feel I have a lack value in life without having this relationship. I often shared my emotion, my doubt to my partner, and the way she responded really comforted me and made me feel that I am valuable.. I am worth.

All participants agreed and accepted that conflicts were part of their relationship dynamics. Conflicts that arose in romantic relationships were considered a vehicle for mutual learning, and an important means to manage expectation and to further validate their values by fulfilling each other's needs. This is shown in the following snippet of the transcript:

> ...my partner is able to help me to calm my emotions.. be a solution for each other's personal needs. (Participant C-07)

Through dating relationships, participants also gain self-existence. When they were valued and considered important by their partner, they felt a sense of existence. A participant, C-06, mentioned that sometimes he felt just her existence was enough to make him feel his existence. This notion was supported by C-03, saying:

> ..there is a feeling of emptiness, lonely, and not worth of love.. I have a friend who felt that he was not lovable material because he cannot afford dating..

Furthermore, C-05, being a Chinese descendent, perceived his existence through the pride status that was maintained through the amount of salary he achieved and the way he kept that information exclusive to his partner:

> As a man, we have a high pride. So anything that is related to pride, that is interrupted, [it] can easily annoy us. For instance, when talking about salary.. I personally said that it was very confidential, and it's non-negotiable to share such information to other people but to our partner.. it is a privilege that one has with their partner.

Another man, C-07, measured his existence through the dominant role he played in making decisions. He mentioned that I would hope that when I made a decision, just go with it and do not make further complaints. Other participants, however, appeared to have a different opinion with him.

It is interesting that, while status appeared to be an important theme, some participants argued that they were not very comfortable with their partner's request to have a photo together posted on social media. This is particularly articulated by C-03:

> It's not that I don't feel that she is beautiful enough.. It's just I am sometimes annoyed with people's comments and reactions to the photos. I just don't feel that it's very necessary to showcase our relationship to public.

Participants also argued that romantic relationships also played a very important role to fulfill their social needs. Although they mentioned that they could have such a social need fulfilled through his community, they believed that it was only through a close, romantic relationship, that they could have a reliable, fulfilling belonging need.

All participants seemed to agree that the presence of a partner is an important factor to increase his sense of self-worth. Participants felt valuable when they had a partner in the context of a romantic relationship.

Theme 2: Relationship as a long-term journey. Participants expected that the relationship that they are involved right now is a long journey. When asked about the end goal of their current dating relationship, only one participant (C-07) who indicated that he did not expect the relationship will end at marriage. With most participants having long-term expectations in their relationship, they endeavored to have clear goals and mutual commitment into marriage.

Conflicts were considered to be part of their investment for the relationship. A participant, C-04, articulated that:

> ..conflict is necessary and healthy... a relationship with no conflict clearly suggest that we are having a bigger problem [than the conflict].. The more conflict that we have, the further we have been going in a relationship, which is a good sign. What is most important is the way we handle it.

His response suggested that his expectation in his dating relationship was beyond for short-term fulfillment.

Another participant, C-05, shared that his motivation for aiming for long-term relationship was inspired by his religious belief. Being a Christian, he believed that having a romantic relationship is a part of God's calling, although he mentioned that some might have different calling to maintain their singleness. He further clarified that "*for me.. I feel that there are many goals that I can better achieve through marriage.*"

Two participants hinted the need for sexual fulfillment as part of their motivation to be in a dating relationship, however none of them mentioned that sex was his primary motivation in dating. In fact, theme around sexuality appeared to be a minor theme throughout the discussion, although a participant (C-06) mentioned that "*Honestly speaking.. I can't deny that sex is important, but it does not explain all.*"

Theme 3: Common societal misconception on men's roles in a relationship. Some concepts around gender stereotypes were discussed and challenged.

First misconception was around how men tended to restrain themselves from communicating their emotions. Participant (C-02) mentioned that:

> I might be different with most men.. but I liked to share how I feel to my partner. It might be an opposite to what currently practiced where men listened to women's talk about her emotion. I must say that I do have such a need and I am enjoying an open communication to my partner, including when I communicate my feeling and she comforts me. I feel okay to share my emotions.

Other participants also in favor of his perception suggested that they agreed that talking about emotion is fine for men. One participant (C-03) even articulated that talking openly about emotion is required for a man to then take a role as a provider of happiness in the relationship.

Regarding the role as a leader in the relationship, participants indicated a rate ranged between 8 and 10 (one participant even rated 11 of 10), suggesting that they believed it was important for a male to be in the leader position in the relationship. Several reasons were justified, including the role of a leader is how a man could contribute in a relationship, being a leader is socially and instinctually prescribed to a man. Nevertheless, participants agreed that being a leader does not necessarily mean making decision without considering or inviting their partner in the process. Hence, the role of a leader would be on overseeing that boundaries are maintained and ensuring that the relationship is directed toward the goals that both parties agree on. In other words, participants valued collaborative work and discussion, while at the same time also expect themselves to be in the leadership position.

Physical standard as the ideal criteria of a partner was also challenged. When asked about participants' consideration in mate selection, they mentioned that the important characteristics are smart, skillful in controlling their emotion, and connecting well with them. A participant, (C-03), shared that:

> I think she needs to tune in with me, so we can communicate well. That's the utmost important because that's what will be satisfying at the end of the day, as when we grow old, sexual need might not be that important.

None of the participants objected to the notion of having a partner with higher career and socioeconomic status than them. C-06, who consistently indicated his position to be of equal role with her partner, even mentioned that:

> I don't see a reason to hinder my partner's opportunity to actualize herself.. If she likes what she does and it drives her to the top of her career, then I am happy with that. For me, the amount of her salary does not make me lower than her because I see her as a person, not the attribute surrounding her.

Another participant (C-05) also mentioned that his current partner has higher educational status than that of his and he was fine with that.

To our surprise, five participants mentioned that they preferred to have partners who were 3–5 years older than themselves, while the remaining two participants did not consider age as an important factor. They cited emotional maturity as an added benefit of dating an older woman.

Lastly, participants believed that it was acceptable for a woman to propose her love to her potential partner. They believed that it did not automatically mean that she was *selling cheap,* unworthy, or had low self-value. Participant C-03 appreciated women's effort to do that as it demonstrated that she was straightforward and assertive, which were desirable characteristics for them.

4 Discussion

Being the first study conducted to explore men's experience in dating relationship from Indonesian perspective, this preliminary study informs valuable insights to better understand what men really think about their romantic relationship from cultural-informed perspective. Interestingly, while sex and power are often quoted as the main themes about how men perceive and expect from a relationship, those themes do not appear to be the predominant topics in our study.

While previous studies have indicated the importance of social status of marriage (Chipperfield & Havens, 2001), and dating, for Indonesian men to their well-being (Himawan et al., 2021b), the present study revealed the specific mechanism to how social status from a romantic relationship accounts for men's well-being. While the existence of a partner is an important determinant to self-prove themselves that they exist, participants in the study also indicated that emotional consequences as a result of having such a status, contributes to their well-being. In other words, participants valued more the quality of the relationship rather than its status. This is evidence through participants' reluctant attitude to have their moment captured on the social media. If the primary need for dating is for social showcase, one might argue that this would perfectly incorporate such a need. On the contrary, participants highlighted the importance of having a reliable source to validate their feelings and belonging needs. Such a finding suggests that men value their relationship quality more than its status and challenged previous research (Chipperfield & Havens, 2001) that considers relationship status to be more important than relationship quality. Therefore, emotional nuance in a relationship is also an important factor to consider in determining men's relationship satisfaction.

Many literatures tend to suggest that attractiveness and short-term fulfillment are the main drivers for men when entering a dating relationship (e.g. Jin et al., 2019). Participants in our group discussion appeared to challenge this idea. In line with the current societal perception of dating as a temporary stage that ends at marriage (Smith-Hefner, 2018), men in this study expect a long-term relationship with their current dating partner. Religious motivation that underlies this expectation was resonated by a participant, suggesting how religion plays an important role for many Indonesian people (Himawan et al., 2022a), including in shaping their relationship experience and expectation. The finding suggests a cultural-informed insight that dating, for many Indonesian men, seems like an important milestone that has a long-term expectation.

Lastly, this preliminary study has set an important ground to understand the Indonesian men's perspective about common social concepts and stereotypes related to gender and romantic relationship. Our finding suggests that men discussing about emotion is not taboo, contrary to the traditional gender stereotype for man (Healey, 2020). Furthermore, it is particularly interesting to explore how hypergamy ideals is negotiated by men in our study. While participants agreed that men should be the leader of the family, they appeared to allow more room for women's participation in the decision making. Such a flexibility is not observed in the traditional role of men where the power seems to be absolutely attached to men (Jones, 2018). While they acknowledge the importance of being a leader, they are more tolerant toward having partners who were older or of higher socioeconomic status than themselves. While this claim needs to be further investigated to increase generalizability power, this notion could pose a solution to involuntary singleness in Indonesia that results from women's misconception toward males' intolerance of her higher socioeconomic statuses (Himawan, 2020).

The study has some limitations. First, the findings might not capture unique experience of individuals with other demographic characteristics that were not possessed by the participants. Considering that ethnicity and religion may play an important role in shaping one's experience in romance, the findings from the study might only represent the majority groups of religion and ethnicity. Secondly, the study was conducted in a city area with high exposure to global and liberal values. It might not accurately reflect perception of men who live in rural areas. Lastly, majority of the participants were in the normative ages for dating. The perception about, and expectation from, a romantic relationship may be different for those who are in the older age groups.

5 Conclusion and Future Directions

Drawing upon the experience of seven Indonesian men, the present study has explored what a dating relationship really means from a cultural-informed masculinity perspective. While many studies around the issues tended to be problematic-based by focusing on the role of men as a perpetrator of interpersonal violence (Antai, 2011; Haselschwerdt et al., 2021; Pratiwi, 2017; Pratiwi et al., 2022; Viejo et al., 2016), the current study endeavors to offer a fresh perspective in approaching the phenomenon that aims to capture different "face" of men in a relationship.

Future studies could investigate the issues by employing participants from different demographic profiles to allow identification of overlapping themes. Since this area receives very little academic attention, future studies should focus on the exploration nature rather than verification of existing theories, to allow an exploration of unique experience.

While further evidence is needed to accurately justify the findings, we hope that the current study could inform valuable insights as an alternative approach to reduce the persistently high rates of relationship problems and violence (Sardinha et al., 2022), by understanding what a man perceives and expects from a relationship through a culturally-informed perspective. An effort to appropriately align perception and expectation from the sides of both genders would then be made possible, which will eventually improve relationship quality.

Acknowledgements We would like to acknowledge the generous participants who voluntarily gave their time to this understudied work. We also acknowledge the assistance of Sandra Sutanto, Giovanni Kaparang, Ester Luvita, Dr. Yusak Novanto, and Princen for their significant contribution in conducting the focus group discussion.

Funding This work received support from the Indonesian Ministry of Education and Culture, Republic of Indonesia, with the grant no: 435/LL3/AK.04/2022.

Conflict of Interest The authors declare that they have no conflict of interest.

References

Antai, D. (2011). Controlling behavior, power relations within intimate relationships and intimate partner physical and sexual violence against women in Nigeria. *BMC Public Health, 11*, 511. https://doi.org/10.1186/1471-2458-11-511

Acocella, I. (2012). The focus groups in social research: advantages and disadvantages. *Quality and Quantity, 46*(4), 1125–1136. https://doi.org/10.1007/s11135-011-9600-4

Bennett, L. R. (2005). *Women, Islam and modernity: Single women, sexuality and reproductive health in contemporary Indonesia.* Routledge. https://doi.org/10.4324/9780203391389

Bloor, M., Frankland, J., Thomas, M., & Robson, K. (2000). *Focus groups in social research.* Sage.

Chipperfield, J. G., & Havens, B. (2001). Gender differences in the relationship between marital status transitions and life satisfaction in later life. *Journal of Gerontology: Psychological Sciences, 56B*(3), 176–186.

Corbin, J., & Strauss, A. (2015). *Basics of qualitative research: Techniques and procedures for developing grounded theory* (4th ed.). Sage.

Fekih-Romdhane, F., Nefzi, H., & Cheour, M. (2022). Relationship between religiosity and sexuality among unmarried male medical students. *Sexologies, 31*(2), 90–98. https://doi.org/10.1016/j.sexol.2021.04.004

He, S. S., & Tsang, S. (2017). Perceived female infidelity and male sexual coercion concerning first sex in Chinese college students' dating relationships: The mediating role of male partners' attachment insecurity. *Personality and Individual Differences, 111*, 146–152. https://doi.org/10.1016/j.paid.2017.02.016

Healey, J. (2020). *Masculinity and male identity.* Spinney Press. http://ebookcentral.proquest.com/lib/uql/detail.action?docID=6034012.

Henao, S., Montemurro, B., & Gillen, M. M. (2022). Exploring the impact of age and relationship status on heterosexual men's discussion of sexuality. *Sexuality and Culture, 26*(2), 449–464. https://doi.org/10.1007/s12119-021-09900-2

Himawan, K. K. (2020). The single's struggle: Discovering the experience of involuntary singleness through gender and religious perspectives in Indonesia. *The Family Journal, 28*(4), 379–389. https://doi.org/10.1177/1066480720950419

Himawan, K. K. (2022). Laki-laki tidak boleh nangis: Pentingnya pendekatan alternatif dalam mengeksplorasi pengalaman lelaki Indonesia dalam relasi romantis. *Jurnal Psikologi Ulayat: Indonesian Journal of Indigenous Psychology, 9*(2), 204–208. https://doi.org/10.24854/jpu712

Himawan, K. K., Bambling, M., & Edirippulige, S. (2018a). Singleness, religiosity, and the implications for counselors: The Indonesian case. *Europe's Journal of Psychology, 14*(2), 485–497. https://doi.org/10.5964/ejop.v14i2.1530

Himawan, K. K., Bambling, M., & Edirippulige, S. (2018b). What does it mean to be single in Indonesia? Religiosity, social stigma, and marital status among never-married indonesian adults. *SAGE Open, 8*(3), 1–9. https://doi.org/10.1177/2158244018803132

Himawan, K. K., Bambling, M., & Edirippulige, S. (2019). Modernization and singlehood in Indonesia: Psychological and social impacts. *Kasetsart Journal of Social Sciences, 40*, 499–506. https://doi.org/10.1016/j.kjss.2017.09.008

Himawan, K. K., Bambling, M., & Edirippulige, S. (2021a). Motivations and reactions to social undervaluation of singles in the married society. *Families, Relationships, and Societies, 11*(4), 569–589. https://doi.org/10.1332/204674321X16316940998258

Himawan, K. K., Underwood, M., Bambling, M., & Edirippulige, S. (2022). Being single when marriage is the norm: Internet use and the well-being of never-married Adults in Indonesia. *Current Psychology, 41*, 8850–8861. https://doi.org/10.1007/s12144-021-01367-6

Himawan, K. K., Martoyo, I., Himawan, E. M., Aditya, Y., & Suwartono, C. (2022a). Religion and well-being in Indonesia: exploring the role of religion in a society where being atheist is not an option. *Religion, Brain & Behavior*, 1–3. https://doi.org/10.1080/2153599X.2022.2070266

Himawan, K. K., Sutanto, S. H., & Pratiwi, P. C. (2022b). Men in romance: A scoping review to explore men's experience in romantic relationships in the patriarchal cultural context. *Manuscript submitted for publication.*

Huang, P. (2017). *"Love" across the strait: Cross-border marriage between Chinese women and Taiwanese men.* ProQuest Information & Learning]. US.

Hull, T. H. (2016). Indonesia's fertility levels, trends and determinants: Dilemmas of analysis. In C. Z. Guilmoto & G. W. Jones (Eds.), *Contemporary demographic transformations in China, India and Indonesia* (pp. 133–151). Springer Cham.

Jin, S. V., Ryu, E., & Muqaddam, A. (2019). Romance 2.0 on instagram! "What type of girlfriend would you date?" *Evolutionary Psychology, 17*(1), 1474704919826845. https://doi.org/10.1177/1474704919826845

Jones, G. W. (2010). *Changing marriage patterns in Asia.* A. R. Institute. http://www.ari.nus.edu.sg/wps/wps10_131.pdf.

Jones, G. W. (2018). Changing marriage patterns in Asia. In Z. Zhao & A. C. Hayes (Eds.), *Routledge handbook of Asian demography* (pp. 351–369). Routledge.

Kalmijn, M., & Liefbroer, A. C. (2010). Nonresponse of secondary respondents in multi-actor surveys: Determinants, consequences, and possible remedies. *Journal of Family Issues, 32*(6), 735–766. https://doi.org/10.1177/0192513X10390184

Langton, C. M., Murad, Z., & Humbert, B. (2017). Childhood sexual abuse, attachments in childhood and adulthood, and coercive sexual behaviors in community males: Main effects and a moderating function for attachment. *Sexual Abuse-a Journal of Research and Treatment, 29*(3), 207–238. https://doi.org/10.1177/1079063215583853

McKeown, J. K. L. (2015). "I will not be wearing heels tonight!": A feminist exploration of singlehood, dating, and leisure. *Journal of Leisure Research, 47*(4), 485–500. Women have more negative stigma than men. Men: bachelor—elevate social status. AGE: singles yang lulus kuliah lebih mendapat tekanan untuk menikah karena lebih mungkin hidup independent and establishing career. Singles yang berusaha (actively trying to get out of singlehood) are less stigmatized.

Powell, R. A., & Single, H. M. (1996). Focus groups. *International Journal of Quality in Health Care, 8*(5), 499–504. https://doi.org/10.1093/intqhc/8.5.499

Sandelowski, M. (2000). Rocus on research methods: Wahtever happened to qualitative description. *Research in Nursing & Health, 23*, 334–340. https://doi.org/10.1002/1098-240x(200008)23:4%3c334::aid-nur9%3e3.0.co;2-g

Sardinha, L., Maheu-Giroux, M., Stöckl, H., Meyer, S. R., & García-Moreno, C. (2022). Global, regional, and national prevalence estimates of physical or sexual, or both, intimate partner violence against women in 2018. *The Lancet, 399*(10327), 803–813. https://doi.org/10.1016/S0140-6736(21)02664-7

Simpson, R. (2015). Singleness and self-identity. *Journal of Social and Personal Relationships, 33*(3), 385–400. https://doi.org/10.1177/0265407515611884

Slauson-Blevins, K., & Johnson, K. M. (2016). Doing gender, doing surveys? Women's gatekeeping and men's non-participation in multi-actor reproductive surveys. *Sociological inquiry, 86*(3), 427–449. https://doi.org/10.1111/soin.12122

Smith-Hefner, N. J. (2005). The new muslim romance: Changing patterns of courtship and marriage among educated Javanese youth. *Journal of Southeast Asian Studies, 36*(3), 441–459. https://doi.org/10.1017/s002246340500024x

Smith-Hefner, N. J. (2018). Courtship and marriage in Indonesia's new Muslim middle class. In R. W. Hefner (Ed.), *Routledge handbook of contemporary Indonesia* (pp. 335–345). Taylor & Francis. https://doi.org/10.4324/9781315628837

Utomo, A. J. (2012). Women as secondary earners. *Asian Population Studies, 8*(1), 65–85. https://doi.org/10.1080/17441730.2012.646841

Vignato, S. (2012). 'Men come in, men go out': Single Muslim women in Malaysia and Aceh. *Social Identities: Journal for the Study of Race, Nation and Culture, 18*(2), 239–257. https://doi.org/10.1080/13504630.2012.652847

Wilkerson, J. M., Iantaffi, A., Grey, J. A., Bockting, W. O., & Rosser, B. R. (2014). Recommendations for internet-based qualitative health research with hard-to-reach populations. *Qualitative Health Research, 24*(4), 561–574. https://doi.org/10.1177/1049732314524635

Perceptions and Understanding of Digital Self-Harm: A Qualitative Analysis of Mental Health Practitioners and Parents of Adolescents

Emily Hickman and Peter J. R. Macaulay

Abstract The proliferation of digital technology has provided considerable connectivity benefits for young people due to the growth of social media platforms and applications. However, there is growing concern regarding the online behaviour 'digital self-harm'. This study explored perceptions of digital self-harm held by key stakeholders—mental health practitioners and parents of adolescents. Semi-structured one-to-one interviews were conducted with five mental health practitioners and four parents of adolescents (aged 11–19 year-olds). Reflexive thematic analysis identified three themes: (a) online power, (b) effective support, and (c) morality and shame. The results suggest that parents and practitioners perceive digital self-harm as a behaviour with a cause and desired effect for young people—a means for adolescents to address power imbalances (e.g., structural, familial, or individual) and express their insecurities. Structured time and open communication are seen as essential for providing effective support for young people who engage in digital self-harm. Digital self-harm is perceived as being morally wrong and even shameful. The findings are discussed in relation to practical implications, especially the need to support parents and practitioners to support young people who may be engaging in digital self-harm.

1 Introduction

In the United Kingdom, Ofcom (2022) reported that 89% of 12–15-year-olds and 94% of 16–17-year-olds have their own social media profile online. There is substantial interest in how such widespread access to and frequent use of social media may affect adolescents' wellbeing and development (Valkenburg et al., 2022). Social media offers opportunities to establish and maintain relationships with peers—a key developmental period for adolescents (Van & Monks, 2020). Whilst the influence of peer relationships on adolescents' behaviours and attitudes has been well-evidenced, most research in this area has focused on face-to-face rather than online interactions (Laursen & Veenstra, 2021; Scholte & Van Aken, 2006).

E. Hickman · P. J. R. Macaulay (✉)
School of Psychology, University of Derby, Kedleston Road, Derby DE22 1GB, UK
e-mail: p.macaulay@derby.ac.uk

P. Macaulay and L. Tan (eds.), *Applied Psychology Readings*,
https://doi.org/10.1007/978-981-99-2613-8_8

The online environment presents many social and recreational benefits. However, one concern is vulnerability to cyberbullying (Macaulay et al., 2022; Zhu et al., 2021). Cyberbullying is defined as the '*wilful and repeated harm inflicted through the use of computers, cell phones, and other electronic devices*' (Hinduja & Patchin, 2015, p. 11). A recent systematic review of cyberbullying prevalence amongst children and adolescents suggests that on average, one in three have experienced cyberbullying victimisation, with one in four identified as perpetrating cyberbullying (Zhu et al., 2021). This suggests an increase in cyberbullying involvement when compared to a previous meta-analysis (Modecki et al., 2014). Cyberbullying victimisation has been associated with negative outcomes such as suicidal ideation and intention (Hsieh et al., 2021), depressive symptoms (Reed et al., 2016), substance misuse (Yoon et al., 2019), and can have an impact on academic achievement and attainment (Hinduja & Patchin, 2015). Furthermore, Marciano et al. (2020) reported in a meta-analysis of longitudinal studies that cyberbullying victimisation constitutes a risk factor for internalising problems. This highlights the negative impact associated with cyberbullying involvement.

Ranney et al. (2020) explored the lived experience of adolescents who have experienced cyberbullying, and revealed that few identify purely as a victim, often taking various roles within cyberbullying such as perpetrator, victim, and bystander. Erikson's (1968) theory of development suggests that identity experimentation is a common feature in the adolescent process of identity formation. However, identity formation in the context of the online environment presents unique challenges, such as a dependence on the perceived social approval from online feedback such as 'likes' (Meeus et al., 2019). For example, Nesi et al. (2018) suggest that unique features of online social media environments create a distinct social context that transforms adolescent peer interactions, affecting the nature of problematic interpersonal behaviours such as bullying. A further feature of online communication is the ability to use it anonymously. Anonymity can be categorised on a functional scale, from 'full anonymity' where users use text-based communication without any identifiable information, to 'pseudonymity' where a user may be represented by a pseudonym or using a fake profile, to 'visual anonymity' (Keipi & Oksanen, 2014; Pfitzmann & Köhntopp, 2001). Such features associated with the online domain highlight how young people can use them to target others online.

Online anonymity has been linked with a phenomenon conceptualised by Suler (2004) as the Online Disinhibition Effect. Suler suggests that people behave differently online than they would offline—they may share more or demonstrate unusual generosity online, in what is termed 'benign disinhibition'; or they may access disturbing content or display aggression online, in what is termed 'toxic disinhibition'. Multiple factors are theorised to interact with each other in creating this disinhibition effect, including minimisation of authority, invisibility and dissociative anonymity. Suler suggests that the anonymity afforded online leads to the separation of 'online self' from 'offline self', which facilitates aversion of responsibility for hostile or deviant online behaviour. This theory has been supported by research which demonstrates an association between toxic disinhibition and cyber-aggression amongst adolescents (Wachs & Wright, 2018; Wright et al., 2019).

These unique features of online communication have contributed to a new form of cyberbullying, referred to as 'digital self-harm'. Digital self-harm is defined as the '*anonymous online posting, sending, or otherwise sharing of hurtful content about oneself*' (Patchin & Hinduja, 2017, p. 762). Studies investigating the prevalence of digital self-harm in the USA and New Zealand suggest a rate of around 6% of adolescents engaging in this behaviour (Pacheco et al., 2019; Patchin & Hinduja, 2017). However, the self-reported nature of prevalence studies raises caution in interpreting these results. Research suggests that this behaviour is more common amongst at-risk young people: those with depressive symptoms, ones who engage in physical self-harm, members of the LGTBQIA+ community, or abusers of drugs and alcohol (Englander, 2012; Pacheco et al., 2019; Patchin & Hinduja, 2017). Furthermore, Meldrum et al. (2020) found a strong positive association between bullying victimisation and digital self-harm. They discuss this association using Agnew's (1992) general strain theory as a theoretical framework and surmise that experiencing a strain (bullying victimisation) contributes to engagement in negative behaviours such as digital self-harm to cope with the negative emotions provoked by the strain.

Digital self-harm has been compared to physical self-harm, with the suggestion that adolescents may engage with it to cause themselves pain in order to experience the positive after-effects they may derive from cathartic emotional release and social validation (Edmondson et al., 2016; Yu, 2021). This idea that digital self-harm may be like physical self-harm in its purpose—a means for adolescents to cope with negative life experiences—is supported by Erreygers' et al. (2022) study which found an association between engagement in digital and physical self-harm. These associations highlight the need for more research into digital self-harm to improve understanding of the behaviour to allow for improved identification and targeted preventative and supportive interventions.

Yu (2021) highlights the roles of both youth mental health practitioners and parents when it comes to identifying and supporting young people engaging in digital self-harm. They suggest that practitioners may be best placed to take a biopsychosocial therapeutic approach to understand motivations and unmet needs of the young person engaging in digital self-harm, as recommended by Beard (2011) in the context of problematic social media use. Furthermore, they suggest that parents play a key role in monitoring, communicating, and signposting their children to support. Parents are encouraged to monitor their adolescent's online activity; however, this presents multiple challenges such as balancing the developmental need for adolescent autonomy with the parental desire to control what their child is exposed to online, and practical issues such as parental lack of technological expertise undermining their ability to set boundaries (Erickson et al., 2016). Communication within the family around incidents of cyber-victimisation has been demonstrated to reduce the psychological impact of these negative events (Hellfeldt et al., 2020); however, young people exposed to cyberbullying report unwillingness to involve their parents in their online conflicts (Young & Tully, 2019).

Parents' role in signposting their young person to support requires an understanding of the point at which they may need to take action, knowledge of support options available, and confidence in other stakeholders such as schools to take the appropriate supportive action—all of which have been highlighted as concerns and barriers by parents (Young & Tully, 2019). When considering problematic online behaviours, parents and adolescents' perceptions around their online risk and the level of parental supervision offered may not be congruent as parents may underestimate their child's involvement (i.e., perceive their child is safe online) and overestimate their awareness of parental supervision (i.e., perceive they are effectively monitoring their child's use of the internet). For example, Barlett and Fennel (2018) suggested a disconnect between parents' and adolescents' perceptions around risk and parental supervision. This suggests that parental perceptions may act as a barrier to providing effective support to adolescents engaging in problematic online behaviours.

This study will address the need for qualitative research on digital self-harm focusing on the perspectives of key stake-holders to better understand the relationship between social media and mental health from the point of view of those working with and supporting young people. It will focus on understanding current perceptions of digital self-harm held by mental health practitioners and parents of teenagers, as these two groups are well-placed to support these young people. This is the first-known comprehensive qualitative study looking at the concept of digital self-harm and exploring the unique accounts of parents and mental health practitioners. Qualitative research allows an opportunity to collect rich and expressive data, whilst thematic analysis is a methodology which is accessible to researchers due to the availability of detailed and comprehensive guidance and has the capacity to produce data-driven themes which are not tied to existing theory (Braun & Clarke, 2006; Coolican, 2019). This study will aim to address the research question: how do parents and mental health practitioners perceive and understand digital self-harm?

2 Method

2.1 Participants

There were nine participants in this study—five mental health practitioners and four parents. In line with Braun and Clarke's (2022) recommendations for consideration of sample size, an exact number was not set, but instead a range of eight to fourteen total participants with an equal split across both groups was aimed for. Following familiarisation of the data by the researcher, the sample size of nine was determined to be sufficient to address the aim of the research by providing rich data from these specific populations. Table 1 describes the demographic information of practitioner participants, and Table 2 of parent participants.

Das et al. (2016) review of mental health interventions for adolescents highlighted that these can be delivered by practitioners in multiple contexts such as online, school-based, or community-based. For the context of the current study, 'mental health practitioner' will refer to professionals employed to support the mental health of adolescents on a digital platform. Mental health practitioners were recruited through the

Table 1 Demographic information of mental health practitioner participants

Practitioner participant	Job title	Age	Gender
Practitioner 1	Emotional wellbeing practitioner	40	Female
Practitioner 2	Clinical training support officer (previously Emotional Wellbeing Practitioner)	41	Female
Practitioner 3	Online counsellor	36	Female
Practitioner 4	Online counsellor/Psychotherapist	59	Male
Practitioner 5	Emotional wellbeing practitioner	38	Female

Table 2 Demographic information of parent participants

Parent participant	Age	Gender	Age and gender of adolescent child or children
Parent 1	60	Male	Female, 18
Parent 2	46	Female	Non-binary, 19 Female, 18 Female, 15
Parent 3	61	Male	Male, 19 Male, 19
Parent 4	30	Female	Male, 11

researcher's workplace (an online mental wellbeing service for adolescents). Practitioners are trained in safeguarding, have robust professional experience supporting children and young people, and have passed an enhanced background check. A total of five mental health practitioners participated in this study, with four identifying as female, and one as male. This gender split is representative of the predominantly female frontline mental health service provision in the United Kingdom (Morison et al., 2014). Their ages ranged from 36 to 59 years.

There are multiple accepted age ranges attributed to the stage of adolescence (Curtis, 2015). For this study, the age range of 11–19 was selected to encapsulate the full range of adolescence and reflect the increase in use of digital technology at this age (Ofcom, 2022). Parents of 11–19-year-olds were recruited through social media platforms. Parents of 11–19-year-olds who worked as mental health practitioners were excluded from participation. A total of four parents participated in this study, with two identifying as female and two as male. Their ages ranged from 30 to 61 years, with the ages of their adolescent children ranging from 11 to 19 years ($M = 17$, $SD = 2.8$).

2.2 Materials

Interview schedules were used to guide the semi-structured interviews. The questions included in the schedules were developed using recommendations from DeJonckheere and Vaughn (2019). For instance, supplementary questions and prompts were employed to encourage expression and gain clarification from participants where needed. All interviews initially explored how participants define and understand digital self-harm. Following this, a definition of digital self-harm by Patchin and Hinduja (2017) was presented to the participant. The interviews then explored motivational factors for digital self-harm, and supportive strategies for young people. All interviews were audio-recorded, transcribed verbatim, and lasted approximately one hour.

2.3 Procedure

Practitioner participants were recruited through the researcher's workplace (an online mental wellbeing community for adolescents). Parent participants were recruited via online advertisement. Those interested in participating were signposted to email the researcher expressing their interest. Potential participants were emailed the participant information sheet detailing the nature of the study and inclusion/exclusion criteria and the consent form. Signed consent forms were obtained from all participants prior to taking part. Consent was also verbally reaffirmed at the start of the interview.

The interviews were conducted online using Microsoft Teams and were audio-recorded. The wellbeing of participants was prioritised, with screen breaks and comfortable seating encouraged and that they may pause or withdraw at any point. The interviews explored mental health practitioners and parents of adolescents' perceptions of digital self-harm. The interview schedule was used to guide the interview, with supplementary questions added to encourage clarification and explanation from participants where needed. At the end of the interview, participants were given the opportunity to ask any questions and were asked how they were feeling post-participation. Participants received a debriefing and sources of support immediately after the interview.

The interviews were transcribed verbatim. Transcriptions and recordings were kept in separate password protected files on OneDrive, separate from the consent forms to ensure confidentiality. Participants' data was anonymised by removing identifiable information from transcripts (such as the name of their workplace) and allocating unique participant codes (6-unit code made up of the first three letters of their surname and the last three digits of their mobile phone number). Ethical approval was granted by the College of Health, Psychology, and Social Care at the University of Derby. Ethical approval was also supported by the digital mental health company involved in recruitment of mental health practitioners.

2.4 Data Analysis

An inducted reflexive thematic analysis was conducted to explore the data (Braun et al., 2014). The flexibility offered in this method allows for the researcher to define the theoretical assumptions used to guide the analytic process rather than them being prescribed as part of a wider methodology (Braun et al., 2014).

Braun and Clarke's (2006) six-stage approach was used to guide the process of thematically analysing the data. A reflexive approach to thematic analysis was employed, acknowledging the researcher's role as an active developer of themes (Braun & Clarke, 2019). The coding process was reflexive and involved immersion in the data through multiple readings, reflection on the codes produced and re-examination of the data. An inductive, data-driven approach was taken when coding the data as the aim was not to apply theory or be guided by previous research but to better understand an under-researched topic like digital self-harm (Braun & Clarke, 2006).

The aim of the analysis was to provide a rich description of the predominant themes, rather than a detailed account of one theme, to gain a broader understanding of the data. A latent approach was taken to the analysis of the data, with the researcher aiming to identify underlying ideas and constructs that influenced the content of the data (Coolican, 2019).

These underlying ideas and constructs were approached from a constructionist epistemological position—acknowledging that knowledge is subjective and shaped by socio-cultural context (Burr, 1995). Rather than focusing on individual experience, this analytical strategy aimed to better understand the socially constructed knowledge that underpinned the perceptions of digital self-harm held by parent and practitioner participants. This approach has been successfully used to understand the perceptions teachers held around the concept of gender (Morrissette et al., 2018), and of self-harm amongst professionals who work with adolescents (Sarubbi, 2005).

3 Results

Three themes were identified from the reflexive thematic analysis: (a) online power, (b) effective support, and (c) morality and shame.

The *online power* theme explores the perception that young people consider themselves to be in a position of power in the online world due to the opportunities for anonymity available to them. Parents discussed how they perceive power dynamics within the family in the context of their adolescent children using digital technology.

Digital self-harm is perceived as a way for 'powerless' adolescents to express themselves and seek support without fear of negative responses. It is also perceived as a representation of a power-shift between the younger and older generations within a family, leading to parents feeling ill-equipped to support their adolescent child.

The *effective support* theme details the challenges and opportunities practitioners and parents identify in supporting young people with digital self-harm. Supporting an adolescent engaging in digital self-harm is viewed by parents and practitioners as requiring communication and time, and they highlight perceived barriers to providing effective support.

The *morality and shame* theme relates to the role that both morality and shame play in understanding and responding to digital self-harm. Parents and practitioners express that they believe a young people's experience and understanding of morality and shame may contribute to their behaviour online. Digital self-harm is seen as something that is morally wrong, with great shame perceived as being attached both to the young person engaging in it and the parent of the young person.

(a) *Online power*

This theme comprised of two sub-themes: the role of anonymity, and family dynamics.

The role of anonymity

Young people engaging in digital self-harm do so by creating and using an anonymous profile to direct abuse at themselves online (Patchin & Hinduja, 2017). Using an anonymous online persona was seen by practitioners as part of a process of constructing an environment where the young person has a sense of ownership and power: '*it's like your anonymous world. You have control to say and do what you want online* via *anonymity'* (Practitioner 1).

This view of the online environment as a different 'world' has been shared by adolescent participants in previous research, where they referred to the online environment as the 'online world' and face-to-face environments as the 'real world' (van der Merwe, 2017, p. 206). A feature of this online world which distinguishes it from the real world is the opportunity it presents to young people for anonymity. Online anonymity is suggested to provide internet users with a further distinction—their 'online self' which can be understood as separate from their 'offline self' (Suler, 2004). This separation between online and offline worlds and identities may result in young people engaging in behaviours online consistent with 'toxic disinhibition' such as cyber-aggression (Wachs & Wright, 2018; Wright et al., 2019). It could be suggested that digital self-harm is a self-directed form of cyber-aggression that is influenced by toxic disinhibition and facilitated by online anonymity.

Parents described the negative responses that can take place when a person expresses insecurities online openly:

> *People put their 'oh feeling cute, might delete later' or 'I don't look that good today', all those malarkey kind of, you know, all of those comments online and then other people are just like 'oh my god. They're just such an attention seeker* (Parent 2)

'Attention seeking' was raised in the above extract as a pejorative term. This response may reflect a perceived violation of a social norm to not seek attention from others. Attention seeking was identified by adolescents as reflecting inauthenticity in Dixon-Ward and Chan's (2022) study, which explored negative responses to social media posts amongst adolescents. Following this, perceived inauthenticity in social media posts was associated with a negative response online amongst adolescents (Dixon-Ward & Chan, 2022). On the other hand, perceived credibility of social media posts sharing self-harm has been shown to influence the level of sympathy, empathy, or sense of injustice the witness feels after reading it (Tan & Chiang, 2022). In the context of digital self-harm, the young person engaging in the behaviour may be using anonymity to express their insecurities—minimising the social risk involved.

When engaging in digital self-harm, the young person can hold multiple roles using anonymity. Practitioners suggested that acting out these multiple roles may give the young person a sense of power and control that they were previously lacking:

> *Maybe the anonymous hurtful comment goes in and they ... as themselves, then put a contradiction in and that maybe makes them feel more powerful? So, they hold multiple roles through the use of anonymity – the victim, the bully, and, in some cases, the defender* (Practitioner 2)

This suggests that the young person engaging in digital self-harm is seen as someone who is feeling powerless. Both parents and practitioners shared their perception that being bullied, feeling isolated, or struggling with low self-esteem may be a risk factor for engaging in digital self-harm. As Mishna and colleagues' (2012) systematic review highlights, prior in-person bullying victimisation is a risk factor for becoming a cyberbully. Furthermore, Meldrum and colleagues (2020) found a strong positive association between bullying victimisation and digital self-harm. This is in line with parents' and practitioners' views for a potential risk factor for digital self-harm.

Practitioners highlighted the anonymity offered by some online support services as integral to the young person's sense of empowerment:

> *the therapist who's wanting to tell, to call the crisis team, she'll go 'no, It doesn't matter. I'll just talk to [online counsellor].' Which I love that she does that because at least she's telling someone... I think that's a big thing for her – that we don't go and tell anyone* (Practitioner 3)

Anonymous online support was described as a '*blank space*' where the young person's words can be heard in '*an absolutely equal forum*' (Practitioner 4). This was contrasted with traditional face-to-face settings such as school, where the hierarchy between teacher and student was seen by some practitioners to be a barrier to the young person's confidence in expressing themselves and expectations around being heard. Whilst Suler (2004, p. 324) frames the minimisation of status and authority through online anonymity as a factor that allows for people to 'misbehave', it may present an opportunity for young people to feel more comfortable to speak their truth and seek support if they are engaging in digital self-harm. The concept of anonymity providing a 'level playing field' for young people amongst adults was highlighted as a positive by young people participating in Keipi and Oksanen's (2014) study.

Family dynamics

Parent participants shared their perception that their teenage children choose what they wish to share with them when it comes to their online use, leading to them feeling powerless in the face of online threats such as digital self-harm:

In reality, you know, uhm, we are clueless, because let's face it, we're only aware of really what our children want to be us to be aware of, aren't we? (Parent 1)

This complements previous qualitative research in which parents describe their 'frustration or resignation' (p. 1398) regarding their perceived lack of control over what their adolescent shares or is exposed to online. Combined with parental feelings of technological inadequacy in comparison to their adolescent children, this has been suggested to contribute to a power-shift within the family (Erickson et al., 2016). In the context of digital self-harm, parents may feel unable to identify the behaviour due to their perception of their powerlessness. Subsequent emotional responses may act as a barrier to effective support or inform future parenting choices.

In response to a young person sharing that they digitally self-harm, some parents expressed their desire to '*deal with it quite strongly using discipline and confiscating their devices*' (Parent 3). This reaction aligns with the belief expressed by some parent participants that digital self-harm is linked with lack of discipline. This perception that lenient parenting may have contributed to, or facilitated, a young person engaging in digital self-harm and subsequent desire to impose an authoritarian parenting style complements the findings of Ferrey and colleagues' (2016) qualitative study. Within that study, parent participants expressed concern that their original approaches to parenting had contributed to the onset of their child's self-harm and so trialled alternative parenting approaches following the disclosure (Ferrey et al., 2016).

(b) *Effective support*

This theme consisted of two sub-themes: communication and offering time.

Communication

Communication around young people's mental health was perceived as challenging by practitioners, highlighting difficulties in explaining digital self-harm to parents of young people who engage in it:

there's that extra challenge of, of saying to, you know, if this is something that the young person wants or needs to be made public to people around them, then like you have to get those, those people to understand that there's an issue here and that could really create another aspect of like, not understanding... 'what, why would they do that? That's crazy why would you do anything like...' (Practitioner 2).

This aligns with the bewildered parental response to self-harm demonstrated in Hughes and colleagues' (2017) thematic analysis. However, this initial reaction is contextualised by Hughes and colleagues as the start of a process of 'sense-making', with the result in most cases being a success in understanding motivations behind self-harm in young people. In the current study, parents could be seen to be engaging with this sense-making process, with most parent participants independently moving from bewilderment (e.g., '*Digital self-harm is just like mind-blowing, I struggle to understand why young people would do that to themselves*' (Parent 4)) to expressing theories and opinions around what could contribute to young people engaging in digital self-harm (e.g., '*young people say nasty things about themselves online as they need help, it's a cry for help*' (Parent 2)).

Understanding the motivations behind digital self-harm was not viewed as the only way to support a young person engaging with the behaviour. The simple act of listening was also highlighted as important:

> *And you don't need to be a professional to just sit and listen to somebody and just for that young person to know that, you know they're loved regardless, they're cared for regardless, and someone's gonna listen to them without judgement, is is is huge, it will have a massive positive impact on the young person* (Practitioner 2)

This relates with a review of the perspectives of young people who self-harm, which highlighted that young people believed that the most helpful way that parents could assist them in managing their self-harm was to talk and to listen to them in a non-judgmental way (Curtis et al., 2018).

Offering time

Young people were seen as spending a lot of their time on social media, with one parent sharing that it '*makes up a huge proportion*' of their child's day (Parent 1). Unstructured time was seen as a risk factor for engaging in digital self-harm, which is depicted by this parent as something that a young person may turn to out of boredom:

> *I imagine that they [young people] would have a difficult time filling their time and they could then drift into into trouble by saying these things online. If they are bored, who knows what they get up to online?* (Parent 3)

Unplanned leisure time was also highlighted as a risk by mothers in Hashemi and colleagues' (2020) qualitative study into preventative strategies to cope with adolescents' online activities. Supporting young people who digitally self-harm to disengage from this behaviour is seen as a process that takes time by parents and practitioners:

> *But it couldn't just happen overnight, there'd have to be steps towards it. You would need to understand the reasons for doing it in the first place before identifying steps to prevent digital self-harm* (Practitioner 1)

Spending time with a young person and listening to them is described as '*investing*' in them by one practitioner (Practitioner 4). A review of perspectives of young people who self-harm revealed that they wish for more love, attention, *time*, support, and care from their parents (Curtis et al., 2018). However, some parents highlighted that this investment of time is a privilege that not all can enjoy:

> *Good parenting is the key, but to do good parenting, it needs time and most parents would say they don't have time ... To a certain extent, we're fortunate that I don't work now, so I'm at home so I have got time to think and look and help ... I dread to think what other people go through in these circumstances who don't have time and have a job and have to go out and can't put any time or thought into it, you know?* (Parent 1)

The financial and practical issues around providing parent–adolescent time were also highlighted by parents of young people who self-harm in Ferrey and colleagues'

(2016) qualitative study. Parents expressed how their desire to spend time at home with their child often conflicted with the demands of full-time work, leading to parental concern both for their child's wellbeing and the financial stability of the family.

(c) *Morality and Shame*

Digital self-harm was perceived by some parents and practitioners as something that is morally wrong or bad. The literature around moral judgement of self-harm suggests that this is a common perception amongst varied social groups such as nurses (Karman et al., 2015) and Evangelical Christian communities (Lloyd & Panagopoulos, 2022). Some attributed young people engaging in digital self-harm to not having the 'right parents' who provide their children with a robust moral education that dictates their future behaviour:

> *if you have the right parents, and you know from a very very early age, right from wrong...then they wouldn't do it [digital self-harm]* (Parent 1)

Shame may also play a part when it comes to supporting a child who has disclosed digital self-harm, with the suggestion that parental embarrassment may act as a barrier to arranging external support:

> *perhaps if parents or guardians feel... perhaps shame, or they're embarrassed by it, they might try and keep it in-house* (Parent 2)

Engaging in digital self-harm is seen as a 'slippery slope', with the risk of blurring of moral lines:

> *it's a very easy transition from kind of like being their own and other people's like victim to to them being the perpetrator of bullying online and, and so I bet it's like trolling, isn't it? I guess it's sort of that, you know you, you, very quickly the lines are very blurred don't you think?* (Practitioner 1)

However, when considered as a choice between bullying oneself rather than directing that negativity at others online, one practitioner suggested that digital self-harm may represent a keen sense of morality combined with low self-worth:

> *I think if you've experienced that [bullying] that's the way that you, you think that people behave. That's the norm for you. But you might you know, you might also have a conscience, so it's like, 'well, I don't want to do that to somebody else, so I'm going to do it to myself because I'm worthless anyway? So I may as well, you know? That's where my focus is going to be. Is on myself'* (Practitioner 4).

This practitioner suggests that young people may attempt to validate the act of digital self-harm as morally acceptable by contrasting it with the bullying of someone else, whom the young person might see as undeserving of such treatment.

4 Discussion

Three themes were identified from the data gathered from interviews with mental health practitioners and parents of adolescents: (a) online power, (b) effective support, and (c) morality and shame. The results suggest that parents and practitioners perceive digital self-harm as a means for adolescents to address power imbalances (whether structural, familial, or individual) and express their insecurities. Structured time spent together, and open communication are seen as essential for providing effective support for young people who engage in digital self-harm. Digital self-harm is perceived within a wider context of morality and as subject to feelings of shame.

Theme 1: Online power

In the *online power* theme, practitioners discussed the role of anonymity. They suggested that the anonymity is necessary to engage in digital self-harm as a means for young people to feel powerful. Online anonymity is seen as key to opening a new 'world' for young people where they feel they are in control. This perception is supported by Suler's (2004) theory of online disinhibition. However, this is not necessarily seen as a negative. Parent participants highlighted that posting insecurities publicly can lead to judgement from peers, who may suspect inauthenticity. Previous research highlights that online anonymity is seen to avoid the social risk involved in interacting publicly as yourself, whilst allowing for positive outcomes such as social validation and self-expression (Kang et al., 2016; Keipi & Oksanen, 2014).

The anonymity involved in digital self-harm may be an attractive option for the young person with low self-worth to express their insecurities whilst minimising social risk. Whether the young person engaging in digital self-harm is considering the risk of being exposed as a self-cyberbully is unclear. Previous research suggests that adolescents perceive that online content is not permanent, and that they are less likely to be held to account for their online behaviour. These two factors have been shown to contribute to the link between anonymity and cyber-aggression towards others (Wright, 2013). Further research is needed on the factors involved in cyber-aggression towards oneself, as in digital self-harm.

Practitioners highlighted that online anonymity allows the young person to take on distinct roles. In the context of digital self-harm, a young person can become the victim and the perpetrator of, and even the intervening bystander to, cyberbullying. This taking on of different identities online was perceived by practitioners to be a means to gain power and control that the young person may have felt they lacked previously due to a low sense of self-worth. Following from this, bullying victimisation may be a risk factor for engaging in digital self-harm, as it is for cyberbullying and physical self-harm (Heerde & Hemphill, 2019; Mishna et al., 2012).

However, from a developmental psychological perspective, taking on different self-presentations can also be attributed to the typical adolescent process of identity formation (Erikson, 1968). There are also other factors which may predispose a person to experiment with self-presentation online, such as narcissism (Mehdizadeh,

2010) or an unclear sense of self (Fullwood et al., 2016). More research is needed into the motivations behind the behaviour of taking on distinct roles within the cyberbullying chain, to better understand digital self-harm.

Practitioners perceived the anonymity offered by some online support services to empower the young person. They described this environment as a 'blank space' where the young person (the talker) was held in equal esteem to the practitioner (the listener). The belief that the online environment allows for a more equal playing field has been termed the equalisation hypothesis, which posits that status is neutralised by anonymity (Dubrovsky et al., 1991). Rappaport (1981) suggests that collaborative approaches which avoid traditional 'helper–helpee' relationships contribute to individual empowerment and positive behavioural change. This perception of anonymous online support as an empowering option was contrasted with the school environment. Practitioners expressed that the power imbalance between teacher and student could act as a barrier to the young person seeking support for any issue.

Within the *online power* theme, parent participants shared their perception that their teenage children hold power over them when it comes to the online world. Parents felt that their adolescents were selective in what they shared with them about their online use, which left them feeling 'helpless'. Discrepancies between parent and child awareness of online threats have been evidenced in prior cyberbullying research, such as Cassidy and colleagues' (2012) study which compared the parent- and child-reported awareness of cyberbullying incidents and found that parent awareness of their child's cyberbullying experiences is low. From a developmental psychological perspective, Finkenauer and colleagues (2002) suggest that the development of secrecy typical of adolescence is key to changes within family power dynamics. It follows that online secrecy could be partially explained by typical adolescent development.

Furthermore, Young and Tully's (2019) qualitative study of adolescents' and parents' responses to hypothetical cyberbullying situations revealed the influence of social norms and acceptability on disclosure to parents. Adolescent participants described beliefs that they would not share cyberbullying experiences in any instance due to peer norms, which require them to keep aggressive interactions within the peer group and not share with parents or other adults. The influence of peer norms and the developmental need for privacy suggests that intra-family power dynamics are not the sole factor in adolescents not sharing with parents. Future research around adolescent online secrecy may benefit from taking an ecological systems approach to better understand the complexities of the interactions between an adolescent's environments and the effect on their online usage (Bronfenbrenner & Ceci, 1994).

In the current study, upon being asked to share what they thought they would do in response to their teenage child disclosing digital self-harm, some parent participants' responses were authoritarian in style—characterised by restriction of devices and decreasing opportunities for independence. This response may be explained by the perception shared by some parents in this study that digital self-harm is due to lack of discipline. Previous research demonstrates that teens are reluctant to disclose online issues to parents due to fear of a restrictive response (Perren et al., 2012). Interestingly, whilst Katz and colleagues (2019) found that a controlling parenting style was associated with a higher prevalence of adolescent involvement in cyberbullying as victims and as perpetrators, they also found that inconsistency within controlling parenting was a risk factor for cyberbullying involvement. They suggest that consistency in online and offline parenting supervision was preferable to avoid contradiction and confusion resulting from different rules across the two settings and subsequent adolescent exploitation of online freedom.

Parent participants in this study referring to themselves as 'clueless' in the face of online threats to their adolescent could be linked with their perception of their ability to monitor their child's online activity. Erickson and colleagues (2016) found that parents who feel technological inadequacy feel frustrated and like 'giving up' in the face of parenting an online adolescent. Martín-Criado and colleagues' (2021) recent study examined the predictive value of variables including parental knowledge of cyberbullying and perception of parental competence in this regard on positive parental involvement in cyberbullying prevention. Their results suggest that perceived parental competence (for example: 'I feel able to detect and identify cyberbullying') is the most influential factor for involvement in parental supervision. The influence of parental knowledge of cyberbullying was highlighted as key to increased perceptions of competence, suggesting that parental education is key to empowering parents to engage with successful online supervision of their adolescents. This may also help parents engage with responding effectively to disclosures of digital self-harm, as mediation parenting strategies have been found to be less effective when parents have low internet skills (Benrazavi et al., 2015).

Theme 2: Effective support

In the *effective support* theme, communication between practitioners, parents, and adolescents was discussed. Practitioners identified communicating with parents following a disclosure of digital self-harm as a potential challenge. They predicted that parents may not understand why a young person would engage in digital self-harm and may react with shock and confusion to a disclosure. This aligns with research around reactions to teenage self-harm disclosures that have found a common response of bewilderment amongst parents (Hughes et al., 2017). It is of note that most parent participants in this study answered that they could not imagine that their adolescent child would engage in digital self-harm, as this may account for a potential reaction of shock.

Hughes and colleagues (2017) noted that parents tended to go through a 'sense-making' process following their initial reaction. Within the current study, parents could be seen to be engaging with this sense-making process, with most parent participants independently moving from bewilderment to expressing theories and opinions around what could contribute to young people engaging in digital self-harm. This suggests that it may be prudent to warn practitioners and adolescents of a potential initial reaction of shock, and that parents may benefit from time and support to digest a disclosure of digital self-harm.

Practitioners highlighted that professional input or training is not necessary to listen to a young person who is disclosing digital self-harm. In previous research, parents have shared that open communication and making a connection with their adolescent are their preferred strategies for mediating their child's internet use (Symons et al., 2017). In Ginott's (1965) seminal work, he suggests that communication is the key factor in a strong parent–child relationship, and that the initial response by a parent to a child's disclosure is often extremely significant to the child. Ginott introduced the idea that active listening is a skill that can be learned by any parent. Some parents in the current study displayed confidence in their existing communication techniques, sharing that they feel inviting their child to talk to them would be a 'normal thing'. However, it is important to consider how the adolescent perceives these communications—in Wisniewski and colleagues' (2017) study, adolescents interpreted parents' responses to disclosures of online risks as 'lecturing'.

The subject of 'time' was raised by parents and practitioners in the current study, under the theme of *effective support*. Parent participants highlighted the 'huge proportion' of their adolescent's day which is spent on social media. Interestingly, Jensen and colleagues' (2021) recent longitudinal study found little evidence to suggest that the quantity of adolescents' daily technology use displaces or disrupts key features of the parent–adolescent relationship on a day-to-day basis.

Social media use can be considered as an unstructured leisure activity, as in Abbott and Barber's (2007) study into the developmental opportunities offered by structured versus unstructured activities. Whilst that study outlined the developmental benefits of structured activity, parent participants in the current study shared their perception that unstructured time is a risk factor for digital self-harm and other harmful behaviour. This view is consistent with the perceptions of mothers in Hashemi and colleagues' (2020) study, who highlighted unplanned leisure time as a risk for problematic online activities. Unstructured time as a risk factor for digital self-harm could be explained by Chapman and colleagues' (2006) theory of deliberate self-harm being motivated by a desire to escape unwanted emotional experiences. Young people engaging in digital self-harm may experience under-stimulation itself as unwanted and uncomfortable, or the unfilled time may present opportunities for unwanted thoughts or feelings to present themselves.

Practitioners highlighted the time commitment involved in supporting a young person engaging in digital self-harm. The word 'investing' was used, implying that those around the young person are expected to give something of their own (their time) to that person to reap the benefits of their investment (the young person's mental health improving or cessation of digital self-harm). Young people who self-harm have expressed their desire for more time with their parents, and a longitudinal study found that self-harming participants reported less frequent contact with their family members compared to those who did not self-harm (Curtis et al., 2018; Turner et al., 2017).

However, parent participants in the current study acknowledged the privilege involved in being able not only to spend time with their adolescents, but also to spend time considering how best to support their child and to reflect. Balancing or juggling caring for children and work commitments is a well-documented concern for parents (Milkie et al., 2015; St George & Fletcher, 2012). The conflict between needing to work full-time and wanting to spend time supporting their child was also raised by parents of young people who self-harm in Ferrey and colleagues' (2016) study. Hsin's (2009) study demonstrated that it was the substance of time spent between parent and child, rather than the quantity, which had the greater impact on child outcomes. However, this study related to cognitive outcomes rather than mental health outcomes.

St George and Fletcher (2012) suggest a solution-focused rather than deficit-focused approach to the issue of time-deficit in working families. In their qualitative research with working parents who have a long commute time, they found that parents placed a heavy significance on 'attentive parenting', which was characterised by parent-led intense moments of connection with their children through shared activities, undivided attention, and mindful listening. As with mediative parenting approaches to internet use, quality adolescent–parent time has been shown to be perceived differently by the parent and the adolescent, with the adolescent's perception being a more significant factor in wellbeing than the parents' (Kutrovátz & Geszler, 2022).

Theme 3: Morality and Shame

In the *morality and shame* theme, the perception that digital self-harm was morally wrong was shared by some parents and practitioners. This fits with previous research around both self-harm and cyberbullying perpetration, both of which have been perceived as immoral (Karman et al., 2015; Lloyd & Panagopoulos, 2022; Young & Tully, 2019). It is unclear whether digital self-harm is being grouped with self-harm or cyberbullying behaviours, and so further research into the contextual positioning of digital self-harm is recommended in order to better understand morality judgements of those supporting young people.

One practitioner situated digital self-harm in the context of cyberbullying and suggested that engagement in bullying oneself online could lead a young person to progress to cyberbullying others. It was suggested that this progression could be a result of 'blurring' of moral lines. This blurring of moral lines may be understood in the context of a process of moral disengagement. A recent systematic review of the literature around cyberbullying involvement and moral disengagement revealed that ninety-one per cent of the studies examining the relationship found a significant positive association between the two (Lo Cricchio et al., 2021). Furthermore, cyber 'bully-victims'—those who are both subjected to cyberbullying and cyberbully others—have been shown to display higher moral disengagement than non-cyberbullies (Arató et al., 2020).

However, the unique self-directed nature of digital self-harm has been interpreted by one practitioner in the current study to be indicative of a strong sense of morality. The practitioner suggests that whilst a bullying victim may perceive aggression towards others as a social norm due to their experience, their personal sense of morality does not allow them to take part in it. Instead, their low self-worth influences them to engage with this norm whilst respecting their own moral code. This behaviour is then deemed as acceptable by the young person by contrasting it with the alternative of bullying another person who they perceive as less deserving of abuse. This could be interpreted as an advantageous comparison—described by Bandura

(2002) as a mechanism used to deactivate negative moral judgements by cognitively restructuring the behaviour.

Parents in Young and Tully's (2019) qualitative study exploring perceptions of cyberbullying shared that they would feel disappointed that their child had strayed from the values they had been taught by bullying others online. This idea that parents hold themselves accountable for their child's morality is complemented by the findings of the current study. Some parent participants expressed their view that adolescents who engage in digital self-harm have not had a robust enough moral education from their parents in their early years. However, parental influence on adolescent behaviour may be wider than initial moral teachings, with poor parenting practice, as perceived by young adolescents, found to be directly associated with higher levels of moral disengagement one year later in Campaert and colleagues' (2018) study.

The phrase 'right parents' was also used by one parent participant. The concept that parents can be 'right' or 'wrong', 'good' or 'bad' as an explanation or response to an adolescent presenting with harmful behaviour has been a theme throughout qualitative research into the experiences of parents of adolescents facing mental health challenges (Berkley-Smith, 2020; Cohen-Filipic & Bentley, 2015; Slemon et al., 2019). The need to assign blame for an adolescent engaging in digital self-harm may be explained by attribution theory, which posits that human beings are driven to assign causality to make sense of the world around them (Weiner, 1995). As noted previously, most parent participants in the current study shared that they could not imagine their adolescent child taking part in digital self-harm. Taken in the context of this behaviour being perceived as immoral, and that a child's behaviour reflects the quality of parenting received, this response could be seen as a defence against moral judgement of their own parenting ability.

Fearing the judgement of others may also act as a barrier to parents seeking external support for their child who is engaging in digital self-harm. One parent participant in the current study highlighted embarrassment and shame around their child's behaviour as a factor in deciding whether to involve others in supporting their child. Embarrassment is characterised as concerning one's public image as it reflects others' perceptions of oneself which do not necessarily align with self-perception—for example 'They will think I am a bad parent'. Conversely, shame often occurs in the absence of others and therefore is suggested to be an emotional representation of an individual's internalised moral judgement of themselves—for example 'I am a bad parent' (Sabini et al., 2001). Shame has been associated with social withdrawal across varied cultural contexts (Sheikh, 2014) and can be explained in the context of social regulation theory, wherein avoiding a perceived negative outcome motivates a person to engage in inhibitory behaviours (Carver, 2006).

It is of note that both embarrassment and shame are highlighted as possibilities in the current study, suggesting that there may be two processes at work—internal and external moral judgements. This was demonstrated in McDonald and colleagues' (2007) qualitative study which sought to understand the experience of parents of self-harming children. Within that study, mothers shared feeling embarrassed when in public with their child due to the visibility of self-harm marks, and also feelings of shame that their child was experiencing extreme unhappiness and engaging in self-harm. Interestingly, the parent participant who gave the most detail regarding feelings of shame and guilt in the current study identified as a woman, and McDonald and colleagues' study involved almost exclusively mothers. Further research may benefit from exploring gender differences in the experience of embarrassment of shame and guilt in parenting adolescents' who engage in self-harmful behaviours.

Self-punishment via digital self-harm was seen by participants as a means for the young person to restore order and address their cognitive dissonance—they feel they deserve pain and so they inflict it upon themselves (Festinger, 1957). This is supported by Stänicke's (2021) recent study which aimed to understand the lived experience of self-harm amongst adolescent girls. A key theme from the analysis of the interview data was 'I deserve pain', which Stänicke suggested formed a self-representation of a person that deserved to be punished. This could be linked back to Patchin and Hinduja's (2017) study, which identified a connection between bullying victimisation and digital self-harm—'I felt like I deserved to be treated that way, so I thought I would get in on the "fun"' (p. 764).

5 Conclusion

In conclusion, the findings demonstrate that parents' and practitioners' perceptions of digital self-harm centre around key themes: online power, effective support, and morality and shame. The online world was perceived to be the young person's domain, where they held power over the family and could feel empowered to express themselves. Supporting young people who engage in digital self-harm includes communicating with involving, supporting, and educating parents to invest time and actively listen to their child. Discussion around the immorality of digital self-harm raised questions around where the behaviour sits in between self-harm and cyberbullying and gave context to both the perceived motivations behind the behaviour and the responses of parents.

Author disclosure statement

There are no competing interests to declare. This research did not receive any specific grant from funding agencies in the public, commercial, or not-for-profit sectors.

References

Abbott, B. D., & Barber, B. L. (2007). Not just idle time: adolescents' developmental experiences provided by structured and unstructured leisure activities. *The Australian Educational and Developmental Psychologist, 24*(1), 59–81. https://doi.org/10.1017/S0816512200029102

Agnew, R. (1992). Foundation for a general strain theory of crime and delinquency. *Criminology, 30*(1), 47–88. https://doi.org/10.1111/j.1745-9125.1992.tb01093.x

Arató, N., Zsidó, A. N., Lénárd, K., & Lábadi, B. (2020). Cybervictimization and cyberbullying: The role of socio-emotional skills. *Frontiers in Psychiatry, 11*(248). https://doi.org/10.3389/fpsyt.2020.00248

Bandura, A. (2002). Selective moral disengagement in the exercise of moral agency. *Journal of moral education, 31*(2), 101–119. https://doi.org/10.1080/0305724022014322

Barlett, C. P., & Fennel, M. (2018). Examining the relation between parental ignorance and youths' cyberbullying perpetration. *Psychology of Popular Media Culture, 7*(4), 547–560. https://doi.org/10.1037/ppm0000139.

Beard, K. W. (2011). Working with adolescents addicted to the Internet. In K. S. Young & C. N. de Abreu (Eds.), *Internet addiction: A handbook and guide to evaluation and treatment* (pp. 173–189). John Wiley & Sons.

Benrazavi, R., Teimouri, M., & Griffiths, M. D. (2015). Utility of parental mediation model on youth's problematic online gaming. *International Journal of Mental Health and Addiction, 13*(6), 712–727. https://doi.org/10.1007/s11469-015-9561-2

Berkley-Smith, R. (2020). *Experiences of Marginalization for the Parents of Children Diagnosed with Mood Disorders* (Publication No. 28021820) [Doctoral dissertation, Capella University]. Capella University ProQuest Dissertations Publishing. https://www.proquest.com/docview/2434742606?pq-origsite=gscholar&fromopenview=true

Braun, V., & Clarke, V. (2006). Using thematic analysis in psychology. *Qualitative Research in Psychology, 3*(2), 77–101. https://doi.org/10.1191/1478088706qp063oa

Braun, V., & Clarke, V. (2019). Reflecting on reflexive thematic analysis. *Qualitative Research in Sport, Exercise and Health, 11*(4), 589–597. https://doi.org/10.1080/2159676X.2019.1628806

Braun, V., & Clarke, V. (2022). Conceptual and design thinking for thematic analysis. *Qualitative Psychology, 9*(1), 3. https://doi.org/10.1037/qup0000196

Braun, V., Clarke, V., & Terry, G. (2014). Thematic analysis. In P. Rohleder & A. Lyons (Eds.), *Qualitative research in clinical and health psychology* (pp. 95–113). Palgrave Macmillan.

Bronfenbrenner, U., & Ceci, S. J. (1994). Nature-nurture reconceptualized in developmental perspective: A bioecological model. *Psychological Review, 101*(4), 568–586. https://doi.org/10.1037/0033-295X.101.4.568

Burr, V. (1995). *An introduction to social constructionism*. Routledge.

Campaert, K., Nocentini, A., & Menesini, E. (2018). The role of poor parenting and parental approval for children's moral disengagement. *Journal of Child and Family Studies, 27*(8), 2656–2667. https://doi.org/10.1007/s10826-018-1097-1

Carver, C. S. (2006). Approach, avoidance, and the self-regulation of affect and action. *Motivation and Emotion, 30*, 105–110. https://doi.org/10.1007/s11031-006-9044-7

Cassidy, W., Brown, K., & Jackson, M. (2012). "Making kind cool": Parents' suggestions for preventing cyber bullying and fostering cyber kindness. *Journal of Educational Computing Research, 46*(4), 415–436. https://doi.org/10.2190/EC.46.4.f

Chapman, A. L., Gratz, K. L., & Brown, M. Z. (2006). Solving the puzzle of deliberate self-harm: The experiential avoidance model. *Behaviour research and therapy, 44*(3), 371–394. https://doi.org/10.1016/j.brat.2005.03.005

Cohen-Filipic, K., & Bentley, K. J. (2015). From every direction: Guilt, shame, and blame among parents of adolescents with co-occurring challenges. *Child and Adolescent Social Work Journal, 32*(5), 443–454. https://doi.org/10.1007/s10560-015-0381-9

Coolican, H. (2019). *Research methods and statistics in psychology* (7th ed.). Routledge. https://doi.org/10.4324/9781315201009

Curtis, A. C. (2015). Defining adolescence. *Journal of Adolescent and Family Health, 7*(2), Article 2. https://scholar.utc.edu/jafh/vol7/iss2/2.

Curtis, S., Thorn, P., McRoberts, A., Hetrick, S., Rice, S., & Robinson, J. (2018). Caring for young people who self-harm: A review of perspectives from families and young people. *International Journal of Environmental Research and Public Health, 15*(5), 950. https://doi.org/10.3390/ijerph15050950

Das, J. K., Salam, R. A., Lassi, Z. S., Khan, M. N., Mahmood, W., Patel, V., & Bhutta, Z. A. (2016). Interventions for adolescent mental health: An overview of systematic reviews. *The Journal of Adolescent Health, 59*(4 Suppl), S49–S60. https://doi.org/10.1016/j.jadohealth.2016.06.020

DeJonckheere, M., & Vaughn, L. M. (2019). Semistructured interviewing in primary care research: A balance of relationship and rigour. *Family Medicine and Community Health, 7*(2), e000057. https://doi.org/10.1136/fmch-2018-000057

Dixon-Ward, K. C., & Chan, S. W. Y. (2022). Faking it': Exploring adolescent perceptions of depression (in)authenticity and 'attention seeking. *British Journal of Clinical Psychology, 61*(2), 177–196. https://doi.org/10.1111/bjc.12339

Dubrovsky, V. J., Kiesler, S., & Sethna, B. N. (1991). The equalization phenomenon: Status effects in computer-mediated and face-to-face decision-making groups. *Human-Computer Interaction, 6*(2), 119–146. https://doi.org/10.1207/s15327051hci0602_2

Edmondson, A. J., Brennan, C. A., & House, A. O. (2016). Non-suicidal reasons for selfharm: A systematic review of self-reported accounts. *Journal of Affective Disorders, 191*, 109–117. https://doi.org/10.1016/.jad.2015.11.043

Englander, E. (2012). Digital self-harm: Frequency, type, motivations, and outcomes. (Paper 5.). MARC Research Reports, Bridgewater State University. https://vc.bridgew.edu/cgi/viewcontent.cgi?article=1004&context=marc_reports.

Erickson, L. B., Wisniewski, P., Xu, H., Carroll, J. M., Rosson, M. B., & Perkins, D. F. (2016). The boundaries between: Parental involvement in a teen's online world. *Journal of the Association for Information Science and Technology, 67*(6), 1384–1403. https://doi.org/10.1002/asi.23450

Erikson, E. H. (1968). *Identity, youth, and crisis* (1st ed.). Norton.

Erreygers, S., Symons, M., Vandebosch, H., & Pabian, S. (2022). Fictitious online victimization: Exploration and creation of a measurement instrument. *New Media & Society, 24*(1), 156–177. https://doi.org/10.1177/1461444820960079

Ferrey, A. E., Hughes, N. D., Simkin, S., Locock, L., Stewart, A., Kapur, N., Gunnell, D., & Hawton, K. (2016). The impact of self-harm by young people on parents and families: A qualitative study. *BMJ Open, 6*(1), Article e009631. https://doi.org/10.1136/bmjopen-2015-009631

Festinger, L. (1957). *A theory of cognitive dissonance* (Vol. 2). Stanford University Press.

Finkenauer, C., Engels, R. C. M. E., & Meeus, W. (2002). Keeping secrets from parents. Advantages and disadvantages of secrecy in adolescence. *Journal of Youth and Adolescence, 31*(2), 123–136. https://doi.org/10.1023/A:1014069926507

Fullwood, C., James, B. M., & Chen-Wilson, C.-H. (Josephine). (2016). Self-concept clarity and online self-presentation in adolescents. *Cyberpsychology, Behavior, and Social Networking, 19*(12), 716–720. https://doi.org/10.1089/cyber.2015.0623

Ginott, H. G. (1965). *Between parent and child: New solutions to old problems.* Macmillan.

Hashemi, S., Esmaeili, M., Ashari, M., & Kazemian, S. (2020). Mothers' protective strategies to cope with adolescents' online activities: A qualitative study. *Preventive Counseling, 1*(2), 13–24.

Heerde, J. A., & Hemphill, S. A. (2019). Are bullying perpetration and victimization associated with adolescent deliberate self-harm? A meta-analysis. *Archives of Suicide Research, 23*(3), 353–381. https://doi.org/10.1080/13811118.2018.1472690

Hellfeldt, K., López-Romero, L., & Andershed, H. (2020). Cyberbullying and psychological well-being in young adolescence: the potential protective mediation effects of social support from family, friends, and teachers. *International journal of environmental research and public health, 17*(1), 45. https://doi.org/10.3390/ijerph17010045

Hinduja, S., & Patchin, J. W. (2015). *Bullying beyond the schoolyard: Preventing and responding to cyberbullying* (2nd ed.). Corwin Press.

Hsieh, Y., Jain, P., Veluri, N., Bhela, J., Sheikh, B., Bangash, F., Gude, J., Subhedar, R., Zhang, M., Shah, M., Mansuri, Z., Aedma, K., & Parikh, T. (2021). Mood and suicidality amongst cyberbullied adolescents- a cross-sectional study from youth risk behavior survey. *European Psychiatry, 64*(S1), S85–S86. https://doi.org/10.1192/j.eurpsy.2021.255

Hsin, A. (2009). Parent's time with children: Does time matter for children's cognitive achievement? *Social Indicators Research, 93*(1), 123–126. https://doi.org/10.1007/s11205-008-9413-6

Hughes, N. D., Locock, L., Simkin, S., Stewart, A., Ferrey, A. E., Gunnell, D., Kapur, N., & Hawton, K. (2017). Making sense of an unknown terrain: How parents understand self-harm in young people. *Qualitative Health Research, 27*(2), 215–225. https://doi.org/10.1177/1049732315603032

Jensen, M., George, M. J., Russell, M. A., Lippold, M. A., & Odgers, C. L. (2021). Does adolescent digital technology use detract from the parent-adolescent relationship? *Journal of Research on Adolescence, 31*(2), 469–481. https://doi.org/10.1111/jora.12618

Kang, R., Dabbish, L., & Sutton, K. (2016). Strangers on your phone: Why people use anonymous communication applications, [Paper presentation]. CSCW '16: Proceedings of the 19th ACM Conference on Computer-Supported Cooperative Work & Social Computing, San Francisco, California, United States. https://doi.org/10.1145/2818048.2820081

Karman, P., Kool, N., Poslawsky, I. E., & van Meijel, B. (2015). Nurses' attitudes towards self-harm: A literature review. *Journal of Psychiatric and Mental Health Nursing, 22*(1), 65–75. https://doi.org/10.1111/jpm.12171

Katz, I., Lemish, D., Cohen, R., & Arden, A. (2019). When parents are inconsistent: Parenting style and adolescents' involvement in cyberbullying. *Journal of Adolescence, 74*, 1–12. https://doi.org/10.1016/j.adolescence.2019.04.006

Keipi, T., & Oksanen, A. (2014). Self-exploration, anonymity and risks in the online setting: Analysis of narratives by 14–18-year olds. *Journal of Youth Studies, 17*(8), 1097–1113. https://doi.org/10.1080/13676261.2014.881988

Kutrovátz, K., & Geszler, N. (2022). Quality time as focused time? The role of focused parental time on the wellbeing of adolescents. *Journal of Family Issues*, Article 0192513X221113857. https://doi.org/10.1177/0192513X221113857

Laursen, B., & Veenstra, R. (2021). Toward understanding the functions of peer influence: A summary and synthesis of recent empirical research. *Journal of Research on Adolescence, 31*(4), 889–907. https://doi.org/10.1111/jora.12606

Lloyd, C. E., & Panagopoulos, M. C. (2022). 'Mad, bad, or possessed'? Perceptions of self-harm and mental illness in evangelical christian communities. *Pastoral Psychology, 71*, 291–311. https://doi.org/10.1007/s11089-022-01005-3

Lo Cricchio, M. G., Garcia-Poole, C., te Brinke, L. W., Bianchi, D., & Menesini, E. (2021). Moral disengagement and cyberbullying involvement: A systematic review. *European Journal of Developmental Psychology, 18*(2), 271–311. https://doi.org/10.1080/17405629.2020.1782186

Macaulay, P. J., Betts, L. R., Stiller, J., & Kellezi, B. (2022). An introduction to cyberbullying. In A. A. Moustafa (Ed.), Cybersecurity and cognitive science (pp. 197–213). Academic Press. https://doi.org/10.1016/B978-0-323-90570-1.00002-4

Marciano, L., Schulz, P. J., & Camerini, A. L. (2020). Cyberbullying perpetration and victimization in youth: A meta-analysis of longitudinal studies. *Journal of Computer-Mediated Communication, 25*(2), 163–181. https://doi.org/10.1093/jcmc/zmz031

Martín-Criado, J. M., Casas, J. A., & Ortega-Ruiz, R. (2021). Parental supervision: Predictive variables of positive involvement in cyberbullying prevention. *International Journal of Environmental Research and Public Health, 18*(4), 1562. https://doi.org/10.3390/ijerph18041562

McDonald, G., O'Brien, L., & Jackson, D. (2007). Guilt and shame: Experiences of parents of self-harming adolescents. *Journal of Child Health Care, 11*(4), 298–310. https://doi.org/10.1177/1367493507082759

Meeus, A., Beullens, K., & Eggermont, S. (2019). Like me (please?): Connecting online self-presentation to pre- and early adolescents' self-esteem. *New Media & Society, 21*(11–12), 2386–2403. https://doi.org/10.1177/1461444819847447

Mehdizadeh, S. (2010). Self-presentation 2.0: Narcissism and self-esteem on Facebook. *Cyberpsychology, behavior, and social networking, 13*(4), 357–364. https://doi.org/10.1089/cyber.2009.0257

Meldrum, R., Patchin, J., Young, J., & Hinduja, S. (2020). Bullying victimization, negative emotions, and digital self-harm: Testing a theoretical model of indirect effects. *Deviant Behavior, 43*(3), 303–321. https://doi.org/10.1080/01639625.2020.1833380

van der Merwe, P. (2017). Adolescent identities in the cyberworld. *Journal of Psychology in Africa, 27*(2), 203–207. https://doi.org/10.1080/14330237.2017.1303129

Milkie, M. A., Nomaguchi, K. M., & Denny, K. E. (2015). Does the amount of time mothers spend with children or adolescents matter? *Journal of Marriage and Family, 77*(2), 355–372. https://doi.org/10.1111/jomf.12170

Mishna, F., Khoury-Kassabri, M., Gadalla, T., & Daciuk, J. (2012). Risk factors for involvement in cyber bullying: Victims, bullies and bully–victims. *Children and Youth Services Review, 34*(1), 63–70. https://doi.org/10.1016/j.childyouth.2011.08.032

Modecki, K. L., Minchin, J., Harbaugh, A. G., Guerra, N. G., & Runions, K. C. (2014). Bullying prevalence across contexts: A meta-analysis measuring cyber and traditional bullying. *Journal of Adolescent Health, 55*(5), 602–611. https://doi.org/10.1016/j.jadohealth.2014.06.007

Morison, L., Trigeorgis, C., & John, M. (2014). Are mental health services inherently feminised? *The Psychologist, 27*(6), 414–416.

Morrissette, V., Jesme, S., & Hunter, C. (2018). Teacher and administrator perceptions of gender in the classroom. *Educational Studies, 44*(3), 295–312. https://doi.org/10.1080/03055698.2017.1373631

Nesi, J., Choukas-Bradley, S., & Prinstein, M. J. (2018). Transformation of adolescent peer relations in the social media context: Part 1—A theoretical framework and application to dyadic peer relationships. *Clinical Child and Family Psychology Review, 21*(3), 267–294. https://doi.org/10.1007/s10567-018-0261-x

Ofcom. (2022). Children and parents: Media use and attitudes report 2022. https://www.ofcom.org.uk/__data/assets/pdf_file/0024/234609/childrens-media-use-and-attitudes-report-2022.pdf.

Pacheco, E., Melhuish, N., & Fiske, J. (2019). *Digital self-harm: Prevalence, motivations and outcomes for teens who cyberbully themselves* (SSRN Scholarly Paper ID 3374725.). Social Science Research Network. https://doi.org/10.2139/ssrn.3374725

Patchin, J. W., & Hinduja, S. (2017). Digital self-harm among adolescents. *Journal of Adolescent Health, 61*(6), 761–766. https://doi.org/10.1016/j.jadohealth.2017.06.012

Perren, S., Corcoran, L., Cowie, H., Dehue, F., Garcia, D., McGuckin, C., Sevcikova, A., Tsatsou, P., & Völlink, T. (2012). Tackling cyberbullying: review of empirical evidence regarding successful responses by students, parents, and schools. *International Journal of Conflict and Violence, 6*, 283–293. https://doi.org/10.4119/ijcv-2919

Pfitzmann, A., & Köhntopp, M. (2001). Anonymity, unobservability, and pseudonymity—A proposal for terminology. In H. Federrath (Ed.), *Designing privacy enhancing technologies* (1st ed., pp. 1–9). Springer.

Ranney, M. L., Lehrbach, K. R., Scott, N. A., Nugent, N. R., Riese, A., Huang, J., Fong, G., & Rosen, R. (2020). *Insights into adolescent online conflict through qualitative analysis of online messages* [Conference paper]. Proceedings of the 53rd Hawaii International Conference on System Sciences, Hawaii, United States. http://hdl.handle.net/10125/64209.

Rappaport, J. (1981). In praise of paradox: A social policy of empowerment over prevention. *American Journal of Community Psychology, 9*, 1–25. https://doi.org/10.1007/BF00896357

Reed, K. P., Cooper, R. L., Nugent, W. R., & Russell, K. (2016). Cyberbullying: A literature review of its relationship to adolescent depression and current intervention strategies. *Journal of Human Behavior in the Social Environment, 26*(1), 37–45. https://doi.org/10.1080/10911359.2015.1059165

Sabini, J., Garvey, B., & Hall, A. L. (2001). Shame and embarrassment revisited. *Personality and Social Psychology Bulletin, 27*, 104–117. https://doi.org/10.1177/0146167201271009

Sarubbi, J. C. (2005). *Demystifying self-harm behavior among teens and adolescents: A social constructionist approach* [Doctoral dissertation, State University of New York Empire State College]. ProQuest Dissertations & Theses Global.

Scholte, R. H., & Van Aken, M. A. (2006). Peer relations in adolescence. In S. Jackson, & L. Goossens (Eds.), *Handbook of adolescent development* (1st ed., pp. 175–199). Psychology Press.

Sheikh, S. (2014). Cultural variations in shame's responses: A dynamic perspective. *Personality and Social Psychology Review, 18*(4), 387–403. https://doi.org/10.1177/1088868314540810

Slemon, A., Jenkins, E. K., Haines-Saah, R. J., Daly, Z., & Jiao, S. (2019). "You can't chain a dog to a porch": A multisite qualitative analysis of youth narratives of parental approaches to substance use. *Harm Reduction Journal, 16*(1), 1–10. https://doi.org/10.1186/s12954-019-0297-3

St George, J. M., & Fletcher, R. J. (2012). Time for work, commuting, and parenting? Commuting parents' involvement with their children. *Community, Work & Family, 15*(3), 273–291. https://doi.org/10.1080/13668803.2012.662802

Stänicke, L. I. (2021). The punished self, the unknown self, and the harmed self–toward a more nuanced understanding of self-harm among adolescent girls. *Frontiers in psychology, 12*, Article 543303. https://doi.org/10.3389/fpsyg.2021.543303

Suler, J. (2004). The online disinhibition effect. *Cyberpsychology & Behavior, 7*(3), 321–326. https://doi.org/10.1089/1094931041291295

Symons, K., Ponnet, K., Walrave, M., & Heirman, W. (2017). A qualitative study into parental mediation of adolescents' internet use. *Computers in Human Behavior, 73*, 423–432. https://doi.org/10.1016/j.chb.2017.04.004

Tan, W.-K., & Chiang, M.-H. (2022). Readers' perceptions of self-harm messages on social media. *Computers in Human Behavior, 131*, 107209. https://doi.org/10.1016/j.chb.2022.107209

Turner, B. J., Wakefield, M. A., Gratz, K. L., & Chapman, A. L. (2017). Characterizing interpersonal difficulties among young adults who engage in nonsuicidal self-injury using a daily diary. *Behavior Therapy, 48*(3), 366–379. https://doi.org/10.1016/j.beth.2016.07.001

Valkenburg, P. M., Meier, A., & Beyens, I. (2022). Social media use and its impact on adolescent mental health: An umbrella review of the evidence. *Current Opinion in Psychology, 44*, 58–68. https://doi.org/10.1016/j.copsyc.2021.08.017

Van, Z. N., & Monks, C. P. (Eds.). (2020). *Online peer engagement in adolescence: Positive and negative aspects of online social interaction.* Taylor & Francis Group.

Wachs, S., & Wright, M. F. (2018). Associations between bystanders and perpetrators of online hate: The moderating role of toxic online disinhibition. *International Journal of Environmental Research and Public Health, 15*(9), Article 2030. https://doi.org/10.3390/ijerph15092030

Weiner, B. (1995). *Judgements of responsibility*. Guilford Press.

Wisniewski, P., Xu, H., Rosson, M. B., & Carroll, J. M. (2017). Parents just don't understand: why teens don't talk to parents about their online risk experiences. In *Proceedings of the 2017 ACM Conference on Computer Supported Cooperative Work and Social Computing* (pp. 523–540). https://doi.org/10.1145/2998181.2998236

Wright, M. F. (2013). The relationship between young adults' beliefs about anonymity and subsequent cyber aggression. *Cyberpsychology, Behavior, and Social Networking, 16*(12), 858–862. https://doi.org/10.1089/cyber.2013.0009

Wright, M. F., Harper, B. D., & Wachs, S. (2019). The associations between cyberbullying and callous-unemotional traits among adolescents: The moderating effect of online disinhibition. *Personality and Individual Differences, 140*, 41–45. https://doi.org/10.1016/j.paid.2018.04.001

Yoon, Y., Lee, J. O., Cho, J., Bello, M. S., Khoddam, R., Riggs, N. R., & Leventhal, A. M. (2019). Association of cyberbullying involvement with subsequent substance use among adolescents. *Journal of Adolescent Health, 65*(5), 613–620. https://doi.org/10.1016/j.jadohealth.2019.05.006

Young, R., & Tully, M. (2019). 'Nobody wants the parents involved': Social norms in parent and adolescent responses to cyberbullying. *Journal of Youth Studies, 22*(6), 856–872. https://doi.org/10.1080/13676261.2018.1546838

Yu, J. (2021). Digital self-harm: A peek into the mind of an online self-aggressor. In M. Khader, L. S. Neo, & W. X. T. Chai (Eds.), *Introduction to cyber forensic psychology: Understanding the mind of the cyber deviant perpetrators* (pp. 67–83). World Scientific.

Zhu, C., Huang, S., Evans, R., & Zhang, W. (2021). Cyberbullying among adolescents and children: a comprehensive review of the global situation, risk factors, and preventive measures. *Frontiers in public health, 9*, Article 634909. https://doi.org/10.3389/fpubh.2021.634909